MW00398586

PRAISE FOR DR
AND *YES, I HAVE HERPES*

A courageous and personal story that I hope inspires and empowers anyone who's felt that there's something wrong with them because of disease. As patient and physician, Dr Loanzon takes empathy to another level.

Dr Larry Burchett MD,
Author of The Gentlemen's Diet

Dr. Sheila Loanzon does an incredible job sharing her personal journey with herpes, as well as educating us on the reality of this prevalent STD. Her book is a page turner, chock full of valuable perspectives like: releasing shame about herpes, communicating openly with sexual partners, and being informed about the details of this STD. I highly recommend her book to anyone wanting to gain a heartfelt and illuminating understanding of herpes. So grateful for her insight!

Juna Mustad,
SEP, Life & Relationship Coach
Co-founder of DailyRelationship.com

It's a rare person who is willing to come out into the open about a shameful secret to help the tens of millions who are imprisoned by it. Not since Kay Jamison's ground breaking and shame freeing, *An Unquiet Mind,* about her "secret" bipolar illness has a book as courageous as Dr. Loanzon's come forth to offer comfort and hope to so many people.

Mark Goulston, M.D.,
Author of *"Just Listen"* Discover the Secret to
Getting Through to Absolutely Anyone

A raw, honest look at something that's been stigmatized for too long. Dr. Loanzon's wisdom will be a great help for teens and adults who are searching for an educated, honest voice at a difficult time. A fantastic resource that I recommend wholeheartedly.

Karin Tanabe
Author of bestselling novels *The Gilded Years,*
The Price of Inheritance, and *The List*

Dr. Sheila Loanzon's startling revelation "Yes, I Have Herpes" kicks-off her candid self-disclosure, astute social analysis, helpful medical advice and unflagging campaign to end shame associated with the diagnosis of herpes. Readers will be captivated by Dr. Loanzon's vulnerability and sincerity, motivated by her enthusiasm and optimism, inspired by her confidence and determination. The message of the book is clear: Herpes is nothing to be ashamed of. Herpes is not the end of a great sex life. Herpes is manageable. Herpes does not define me. Your view of herpes will be forever changed as you share her remarkable journey.

Sonja T. Van Laar, Ph.D.

Licensed Clinical Psychologist., Women's Health Services

Yes, I Have Herpes

Yes, I Have Herpes

A Gynecologist's Perspective In
and Out of the Stirrups

DR. SHEILA LOANZON, DO

Disclaimer:
The information provided in this book is designed to provide helpful information on the subjects discussed. This book is not meant to be used, nor should it be used, to diagnose or treat any medical condition. For diagnosis or treatment of any medical problem, consult your own physician. The publisher and author are not responsible for any specific health or allergy needs that may require medical supervision and are not liable for any damages or negative consequences from any treatment, action, application or preparation, to any person reading or following the information in this book. References are provided for informational purposes only and do not constitute endorsement of any websites or other sources. Readers should be aware that the websites listed in this book may change. The author has no financial relationships to disclose.

Names and identifying details of patients and individuals are fictitious or have been changed to protect the privacy of individuals.

DEDICATION

This book is dedicated to my scared 20-year-old self. If she could see the person that I have blossomed into 16 years later she would be so proud and feel safe. She is the sacred person I write this for.

CONTENTS

ACKNOWLEDGMENTS

You chose.
You chose.
You chose.

You chose to give away your love.
You chose to have a broken heart.
You chose to give up.
You chose to hang on.

You chose to react.
You chose to feel insecure.
You chose to feel anger.
You chose to fight back.
You chose to have hope.

You chose to be naïve.
You chose to ignore your intuition.
You chose to ignore advice.
You chose to look the other way.
You chose to not listen.
You chose to be stuck in the past.

You chose your perspective.
You chose to blame.
You chose to be right.
You chose your pride.

You chose your games.
You chose your ego.
You chose your paranoia.
You chose to compete.
You chose your enemies.
You chose your consequences.

You chose.
You chose.
You chose.
You chose.

However, you are not alone. Generations of women in your family have chosen. Women around the world have chosen. We all have chosen at one time in our lives. We stand behind you now screaming:

Choose to let go.
Choose dignity.
Choose to forgive yourself.
Choose to forgive others.
Choose to see your value.
Choose to show the world you're not a victim.
Choose to make us proud."
— Shannon L. Alder

I would like to thank Julien, my life coach, who piece by piece gently opened me to the realization I am perfect just as I was created. To have someone who is genuine, sensitive, full of love and gifts is a true blessing for which I am eternally grateful. I never would have become the woman I was meant to be without your guidance. Your updraft has carried me higher than I could have ever flown on my own.

I would like to acknowledge my past partners for giving me the experiences which enabled me to grow. I am grateful to them, however harsh the lessons may have been. At the time, the part of me that felt anger, abandoned, betrayed, and criticized rose to the surface and the woman who has stepped out of these ashes has transformed out of these experiences into her greater self. Please forgive me for the way I acted toward you.

I wholeheartedly honor the light and love of my friends and family for their support and openness. Sharing this diagnosis has been emotional; however, I discovered I was hardest on myself. I overflow with generous and abundant love and enjoy moving forward in this world, completely open and honest with my loved ones. Thank you, Jaime, Broyo, and Tory for ferociously supporting my great vision. My gratitude to Jen, your late night edits and suggestions saved me!

Thank you, Alicia, for your guidance and expertise while writing my book. Your work is awe inspiring, and none of this could have come to fruition without you! To my mermaids who taught me to boldly share in a room full of receptive strangers and yoga/ Pilates/ WeCare retreats who gave me breath, awareness of my body, and detoxification: Thank you for the exploration and clarity I gleaned with you in the past two years. You have been preparing me for this exact moment.

To my partner, Dan, who supports me through this writing process, accepts me exactly as I am, views our relationship in positivity and light, and loves me unconditionally. I have been working all my life toward someone like you, Baba.

INTRODUCTION

"Self-care is never a selfish act—it is simply good stewardship of the only gift I have, the gift I was put on earth to offer to others."

— Parker Palmer

MY NAME IS Doctor Sheila Loanzon, and I am a practicing, board-certified obstetrician and gynecologist. I am a Diplomate of the American Board of Obstetrics and Gynecology and a Fellow of the American Congress of Obstetrics and Gynecology. Being five years out of residency at the time of this book, my practice has grown to approximately 3,000 patients, with an average of 20-25 patients a day. My office day is a combination of obstetric and gynecologic patients where diagnosis, treatment, and counseling of general women's health occurs. Proudly, I have one of the highest visits per day of providers in my office.

As a professional, I provide my patients with reassurance, education, and management of medical diseases without judgment. This safe office environment creates space for a patient to confide in their physician what she would prefer to hide. Specifically, I pride myself on educating and reassuring patients; I like being the person who can inform them from a professional perspective. Connecting with my patients is important to me, and I began to realize that my unique understanding of patients was an opportunity to create depth due to my own gynecologic history.

I am qualified to write this book because I was diagnosed with herpes when I was 20 years old. A mere pre-med sophomore in college, I ignored and hid it for 10+ years, and I have just recently started sharing my diagnosis with partners. Through my own story, I would like to expose my own mistakes, lead by example, and re-empower women, showing how to transition forward with herpes to lead a healthy emotional, physical, and sexual life.

If you contract genital herpes, you are naturally concerned about how it will impact your overall health, sex life, and relationships. Your doctor may be the first person you turn to for support, and is an important resource. Though I feel physicians are excellent at giving a diagnosis based on the clinical picture, most do not have the time in the office to educate or counsel their patients fully. Because of this, patients may feel very alone with their diagnosis and often the support system desired is not there.

Writing this book is not only a way for me to share through my own story but is also a vital contribution to the resources available on herpes for the lay-person. Women's health issues are not just about abnormal pap smears, birth control, pregnancy, hormones, and menopause; equally important are a woman's self-image and self-care. My hope by creating this book and sharing my experience is to help others find confidence, self-worth, and acceptance within the herpes diagnosis.

Herpes has a huge stigma in our culture due to its sexual acquisition. My decision to share my experience with others comes from the fact that I have the unique position of being both the professional and the patient. I understand the personal challenges of herpes, while also having deep professional knowledge of the virus. If I can help at least one person feel they are not alone, then this endeavor will be worth it. There is a plethora of information on the Internet for non-medical professionals and research studies published in medical journals, but a personal perspective is something unique. I will have succeeded if I can empower women with the knowledge that they are not alone and can overcome self-judgement and create healthy sex lives moving forward.

This book is for the vulnerable women:

- Who fear herpes.
- Who fear they are going to be left by their present or future sexual partners.
- Who feel victimized and want to understand what has happened to their bodies.
- Who desire to love themselves again.
- To demystify herpes for themselves and then explain herpes clearly to their partners.
- Who question their self-worth and feel the disease has taken self-worth away from them.
- Who feel like they are outcast because of their difference.
- Who have a secret they want to share and cannot find the words.

I believe this book can also be helpful for any partner wanting to understand more about the virus and desire to empathize with their partner's journey. This book is also applicable to men and for anybody who has any sexually transmitted disease causing self-worth and self-love issues.

Most important, this book is for the young woman I was at 20 years old, for the person I have transformed into today, and the flourishing woman I connect with in my future. I lead by beginning with the end in mind, and I write this book for you.

Chapter One

SHIFTING PERSPECTIVE: MY STORY

"Out of your vulnerabilities will come your strength."

— Sigmund Freud

A S AN INVINCIBLE 20-year-old sophomore cheerleader in college, I began dating Patrick, my first real boyfriend. The decision to "save myself" until I was older was not a religious decision or out of respect for my upbringing, I had just not met the right guy to blast through that end wall of sexuality I considered to be vaginal intercourse. We dated several months and became best friends before delving into a physical relationship.

The thought of having vaginal sex seemed daunting to us both as he was a virgin, too; so we decided to enjoy other sexual activities until we felt comfortable. It was a few days after having oral sex that I noticed it was so exquisitely painful for me to urinate that I cried and feared going to the bathroom. It seemed a little bit more painful than a urinary tract infection, so I took a mirror (which I had never done before) and peered below. My heart pounded as I noted small sores on both sides of my labia. I immediately went to the school nurse, who took a painful culture of the sores and started me on antiviral medication. She explained simply that we had to wait for the culture to come back, scribbled a prescription, and with a swift tear of the prescription pad, promptly left the room with me covered in a paper sheet, freezing and pondering what the hell just happened.

I did not blame Patrick at the time. I was just confused and scared that I had done something bad. I went to the cafeteria, where my girlfriends were eating, and when they asked me, "What's going on, did you have to go to the campus clinic?" I said, "I have some bumps down there. I went to the nurse practitioner who gave me some antibiotics, and we're just going to wait and see." Neither I nor the nurse used the word "herpes." A few days later, the campus nurse called and confirmed the diagnosis was herpes. Looking back now as a clinician who diagnoses patients, I do not remember her giving me counseling or safe sex practice guidelines regarding herpes. I do remember feeling brushed off and considered a closed case in her files.

When I spoke to Patrick about it, he said, "I've never had anything down there." And I said, "Well, she says that I could have gotten it from a cold sore," to which he replied, "I get cold sores on my lip all the time, but I don't have any now." Then I said, defeated, "Well, I guess that's how."

I took my medication as prescribed and hoped the topic would disappear, similar to when my outbreak cleared without a trace. A close girlfriend once followed up asking casually, "Hey, how's that bump down there?" and I brushed her off admitting, "It's fine. It's fine; it's nothing." I never blamed Patrick for not knowing he could pass this to me. We entered into the relationship naive and equally.

I felt embarrassed, shameful, and alone. I viewed myself as perfect until then—my immigrant parents' golden child with the bright smile, sparkling personality, and physician future, as well as their hope for a better life than the Filipino homeland we came from. I did not want to believe I had an incurable diagnosis; instead, I swept the subject under the rug and pretended it never happened.

Luckily, I had such sparse outbreaks throughout the years that followed that I actually did forget I had herpes. Patrick did not have any genital outbreaks. I dated him for 1.5 years, and when we broke up, I did not feel the urge to blab about what he gave me. I preferred to internalize and defuse within.

I did not have many sexual partners afterward, but admittedly, I did not tell my partners. If and when I ever did have an outbreak, I was cautious to avoid intimacy at that time. Condoms were used regularly. None of my other partners said they developed lesions, so I considered myself lucky. Back then, I did not allow myself to truly understand the gravity of the diagnosis. In retrospect, I believe that would mean that I would have to change my thought process of who I am.

During my third year of medical school at the age of 24, I met my first husband, Seth, a 33-year-old doctorate student. The very first time we were together, approximately one month into the relationship, we had unprotected sex. I did not have an outbreak at the time, but we got carried away in the moment. We had believed we were each other's "The One," so it did not seem like a poor decision. The next day, I casually mentioned, "That was so crazy what we did last night ... but it doesn't matter; it's not like you have an STD[1]." We had never had an STD discussion before being sexually intimate, and he shrugged, got quiet, said "Nope," and turned around.

He came back to my apartment about a week later and had this very sullen look on his face. He walked in, sat on the couch, and said, "I just have to be very honest with you." He broke down, crying hysterically, and through tears told me that he had a diagnosis of herpes. He said that he did not have an outbreak at the time and things were just happening so quickly, we were caught up in the moment, and he chose not to tell me.

---

[1] STD= Sexually Transmitted Disease.
STI= Sexually Transmitted Infection.
STIs are infections that are commonly spread from person to person through sexual contact. STD and STI are terms used interchangeably in this book.

He had been talking to his best friend about the dilemma and, because he liked me so much, she urged him to be honest.

In the brief seconds while Seth waited for my response to his monstrous admittance, I had an eternity of a conversation in the back of my mind, wanting the scream out to him, and the world, "We are twins! I HAVE HERPES, TOO!!!" This was my opportunity, and I was on the brink teetering between one choice or another. Do I join him in his community and identify as also having herpes? Or do I choose the role of the victim and allow him to believe that he did this to me?

I was afraid that he was going to leave. I was afraid he was going to judge me for not being honest. I wanted him to feel punishment for not being honest with me, and in a way, punish myself. I wanted him to be indebted to me so he could never leave me. I wanted to be a victim. I did not want to embrace a diagnosis that I struggled to accept.

I let the moment pass in silence. I looked him in the eye, quietly soothed, and chose my stance. "It's okay, we will get through this together," and climbed into his lap and let him sob on my shoulder. At the time, I felt he could be my new perfect life and having a partner who gives me herpes is what I am destined to have.

Two weeks later, I had my "first" outbreak. At this point, I had gone through the first two years of medical school, which teaches academic diagnosis, etiology, presentation, and treatment. One day, while Seth was rushing out the door for work, I informed him, "I think I have an outbreak," pretending that it was my first time, pretending to be scared. Perhaps he did not know how to cope or maybe he was too busy with work, but he just said, "I can't talk about this right now; I've got to go." I remember thinking: please walk me through it, be my partner, and give me some reassurance. Instead, he walked out the door, saying "I gotta go."

I took myself to a gynecologist, who confirmed my diagnosis. I started antiviral medication and went through the outbreak alone. Seth and I never discussed herpes again. He did not tell me if he had outbreaks, but I decided to take Valacyclovir suppression medication to decrease flare-ups. He took it only a few months, at my request, but I took it faithfully for two years to commit to managing my STD life.

Seth and I eventually ended up divorcing for non-related reasons. The lead up to the end was approximately six months, during which time we began distancing and growing apart. He declined going to marriage counseling together. He was seeking counseling for his own issues, and I was going to my own psychologist to soften the blow of what was transpiring in our relationship. It was May 2010 when Seth and I sat down to dinner and he asked for a divorce. He felt that when he married me, he married for selfish reasons: he had a fear of abandonment as he was left as a child and did not want me to leave him. At this time in his life four years later, he wanted to divorce me for selfish reasons as he felt we could never fully connect. He desired that emotional connection.

I flashed back to the first discussion on the couch and thought: Did we never connect because I did not admit my herpes diagnosis to him? Or is it because he never wanted to talk about his childhood and abandonment issues? We were sitting at the dining room table, and I saw myself crying on the floor, begging on my knees, asking him not to leave me. A strong voice in my head struck me at that moment, "I am Sheila, I don't beg!" I brushed my knees off, blew my nose, wiped my eyes, and asked how we were going to separate our shared items.

I was divorced and graduated from residency at 30 years old. I moved back to my home state and began work as an ob-gyn attending in a large multi-specialty practice. For two years, I focused on my career and recovered emotionally from the divorce. When I started dating, I noticed I was attracting the same type of gentleman. I was choosing men whose facade was presentable to myself, colleagues, and family, but deep down were lying to themselves, cheaters, or were emotionally immature.

After my third dating disappointment in a row, I finally got tired of feeling like the rug was constantly being pulled out from underneath me. I sobbed to my close girlfriends that it was like going to the beach and standing amongst waves that kept knocking me down over and over. I was beginning to feel that I did not have the strength to get back up again. I decided to make the commitment to myself to do internal work as I felt there was a common thread in all of the relationships—it was ME! I met Julien Adler through a mutual friend, whom I had witnessed make dramatic transformations in her relationships, partners and family specifically. Julien and I began our work in January 2014, and I trusted in his process.

MOVING FORWARD: IN LIGHT AND IN LOVE (OCCASIONALLY IN DARK AND IN DISLIKE)

"It is not what happens to you that measures who you are; It is how you choose to respond that does."

— Julien Adler

It took approximately one year of working with Julien and attention on core values such as self-love and self-worth to build my confidence. Ultimately, I was able to shift my perspective that if a gentleman I was dating did not want the possibility of acquiring herpes, I could leave and find another phenomenal guy who would find me a stunning goddess catch.

It took nine months of soul searching and intense exercises to grow in love with myself. I joke with friends that I was asexual at that time, but when it was time to date, a gentle suggestion from Julien was to abstain from attaching to a new partner immediately. I was changing and growing so rapidly as I cleared family, cultural, religious, and pop culture patterns and truly relied on myself. Any partner that I invited into my life would have been outgrown in a short amount of time.

In my sessions, I discovered large parts of my life that were incompatible and giving me angst. Herpes was part of my identity that I was denying and shying away from. I was afraid—I wanted to look perfect for my partners, family, and colleagues. I wanted people to like me, but this disease was in the background, hanging over my head. I lied for years by not telling my sexual partners and was subconsciously ashamed of my deceptive behavior. I was terrified to confront my partners and felt shame in the 15 years of nondisclosure.

But how could I break the cycle? Could I possibly admit something shameful about myself without the self-confidence to stand on my own if they left me? If my partner did leave me after knowing my diagnosis, would it prove what I felt about my self-worth at the time—that I was not worth sticking around for? I know how to repetitively survive relationships when a guy cheats on me or treats me poorly. I know that scenario pattern. Could I survive something I am not familiar with? Would I be judged by my profession and peers for being a moral physician but also a normal scared human being with fear and emotions?

After years of secrecy, it became clear it was important for me to tell my partners, and that is ultimately how this book came about. My strategy before was to be quiet and ignore the disease in hopes that herpes would go away and cease to exist for me. In other aspects of my life, I was so very open that it did not make sense for me to withhold my whole truth. It is exhausting to have a mismatch of external confidence but internal weakness.

Chiefly, I wanted to be congruent where the inside matched the outside so I could live my life with integrity.

I felt comfortable and confident to start dating after a few seemingly simple exercises that Julien had me complete. The effect on me was monumental and exponential. I believe I have had the successes I have had because I did the internal work. The process was difficult and frustrating but well worth it. I have included these exercises later on in the book (please refer to Sheila's Self-Love Bootcamp p. 98)

My Pivotal Partners

Brian was an executive I had been set up with by a friend. He was funny, intelligent, well-traveled, and enjoyed similar activities as me. We had been dating for a month or so when our relationship began becoming more sexually charged. I was in a critical part of my work with Julien, teetering between fully expressing myself and clinging to my past patterns of settling into a relationship too quickly, and not honestly informing my partners about herpes. I successfully managed to avoid sex one afternoon; however, on the phone later that night our conversation ended up there. Brian was expressing how grateful he was to be 39 years old, never got a girl pregnant, and had survived his 20s without getting an STD. It is ironic that the situation you want to avoid just pops up in normal conversation! I was petrified to speak but knew my time had come.

I took in a big breath of air and stuttered slowly, with my voice cracking and tears in my eyes, "I feel like we're heading in this particular direction, and I just have to be very honest with you. #1: I'm not ready to become more serious with you. I have this past I'm working through, and I don't think it's the right time for me to settle down. With sex comes feelings for me, and I'm not ready. But more important, #2: I have herpes. I haven't had an outbreak in a while. My previous partners have never had an

outbreak, but this is something that I think I should tell you. I
understand if you need some time to think about it but please
just let me know when you arrive at your decision." He took a
deep breath in, became silent, and stated that he appreciated
my honesty and would like the night to think about how he
wanted to proceed.

iMessage with ▮▮▮▮▮▮▮
7/18/14, 5:58 AM

> Hi Sheila, I have to admit that I have been quite torn since
> our conversation last night. On the one hand, I really enjoy
> your company and honestly believe that we would have a
> lot of fun together. On the other hand, it's pretty clear that
> we are in different spots in terms of what we want
> relationship-wise. I really would like a committed
> relationship with long-term potential. What I heard from
> you is that you need some time to learn to date and break
> some of those old patterns.
> Unfortunately the latter is outweighing the former right
> now. Even though I know how enjoyable it would be to
> continue things, I also realize it would be doing a
> disservice to both of us given that you just aren't ready for
> that. So with that said, I think we should put things on
> hold for at least a few months until you've gotten past this
> period of no exclusive relationships. If neither of us are
> dating anyone at that point, perhaps we can reconnect.
> Would that work for you?
> Btw, I forgot to mention that I really appreciate and
> commend your openness and honesty with me last night.
> Although I am fairly certain it is not what you wanted to
> hear, your candor prevented us from going down a path
> that you most likely aren't ready for.

I was distraught by Brian's response but I was also proud of
myself for gathering up courage to admit to a partner before
becoming sexually active. The sting from his choice to not move
forward with me was calmed by my one grand step forward.

Ben was my intellectual equal. He was witty, friendly, and had
an admirable educational pedigree and a boisterous personality.
Our first date lasted 8 hours, which included 2 hours of playing
duets on the piano and singing. I instantly felt comfortable with

him; our conversations could easily last over 12 hours in one sitting with both of us talking and sharing. We had been sitting on the couch cuddling, and I felt inclined to admit to him that I have herpes. He admitted that he knew some things about it, but not a lot. He was medically inclined and wanted to do his own research. I cried when I got into the car. I cried over proudly admitting I had herpes, I cried over breaking my own heart, and I cried because this great guy may pass me over.

The next day, Ben texted me something silly, which was reassuring. He let me know a week later when he invited me to a sushi lunch, "I did my independent research and talked to a few people. It's interesting, as much as I have gone through life being with other people, it never occurred to me that I was more worried about pregnancy than STDs. Acquiring herpes makes me nervous but I like you. I would like to see where our dating goes, but how about we put the physical activity on the back burner for now. If you could please take the suppression medication to protect me in case we move forward, that would make me feel a lot better."

I was reassured and it felt like we had the opportunity to go back to dating, like in high school. Just getting to know each other! Dating Ben was a very freeing moment and a gigantic celebrated leap forward. I appreciated that he gave me the safe space to fully express myself. We dated for three months before I felt we were not the right fit for lifelong partnership and thus I ended the relationship. If we had reached the level of intimacy of having intercourse, I believe our connection would have been so much stronger because of my honesty and his understanding. It would have been an environment for deeper intimacy. He remains a great friend!

My truly pivotal moment came while I was dating **Sebastian**, a suave divorced 41 year old who ran a large Bay Area sports

SHIFTING PERSPECTIVE: MY STORY • 11

company. We had actually been dating for about three months, and I felt we were moving in the right direction. He would contact when he was traveling abroad on vacation in Switzerland and had a European finesse, maturity, and grace about him that I admired. We had started to be intimate but used condoms. When I was at his home, there were certain things that I thought were off. I observed that his mail and his individual cable setting was in a different name. When I mentioned the discrepancy, he explained to me that he used his formal Swiss name on his bills and Sebastian is what he used with online dating because with a few details his company and worth was discoverable.

While he was abroad, I "Google stalked" him (I do not recommend doing this, in medicine or in dating!) and found that, in fact, he was 10 years older than he had stated! I debated whether or not to reveal his big secret when he returned, but decided that I was having fun exploring the Bay Area with him, and we were still in the discovery stage of dating.

As time went on, I became more upset that Sebastian was not admitting to his insecurities. But how could I be hypocritical? He was directly reflecting exactly what I was doing! I began to compare how a few weeks earlier with Ben, I was able to express myself so clearly, and with this dating experience, I wanted to hide. Subconsciously, this relationship invoked different actions and the desire to protect my insecurities. Interesting!

Confiding in him in person would have been the most powerful position to be in so I could observe his raw emotions. I was mentally preparing for his anger and attempting to respect his reaction. I wanted to have ownership of the situation because I ended up creating it. If Sebastian gets angry, it was his prerogative and right to have his emotional response.

However, due to work schedules, the opportunity arose to tell him over the phone, and I did not waste any time starting the conversation. Assuredly, I stated: "Sebastian, I am really enjoying getting to know you, and I am interested in moving forward. I have not been honest with you, and I want you to know that I have herpes. We have been careful but I want to be honest so we can hopefully move forward together. I apologize for not being forthright with you; I do hope you can forgive me." He took a deep breath, gracefully replied with that old European air that he appreciated my honesty, and he would have to think about it. I told him I would give him the space and time he needed. Simultaneously, I grappled with exposing his age after my research, but after checking my gut, I realized that this opportunity was not about uncovering someone else's insecurity, but facing mine. We proceeded to have a pleasant 45-minute conversation afterward, and then I waited to hear from him.

Sebastian contacted me several days later via text:

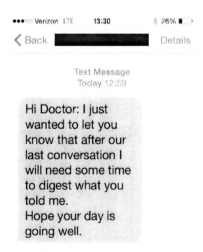

I did not hear from Sebastian again, and I was surprisingly well adjusted with that. From this experience, I learned there are so many layers of trust and, equally, there are many layers to the truth. We can trust people to take care of our cat, and we can trust people to pick us up from the airport, but there are certain people who we would not trust with our banking information. This does not invalidate the other types of trust. However, often when someone causes a loss of trust in one domain, suddenly all trust can be lost. Just like a hallway of truths, we have different levels of doors that we allow others to pass through with entrance at different times. For me, the herpes door was closed to Sebastian until I was ready to open it; to me, his true age was a coveted door he wanted to restrict and keep closed.

Dan is the gentleman I am currently dating who is a 41-year-old real estate development director whom I met online and with whom I had an instant connection. We became friends first, which is an experience I have never had dating before in my adult life. Perhaps it was the one month of chatting on the phone and texting before our first date (our work schedules were so busy at that time we could not meet in person!) With Dan, it is easy for me to express myself; he is wonderfully patient, emotionally mature, nurturing and creates a safe space for me, despite some of my lingering insecurities. When I met Dan, I was at the point in dating that if things did not work out with this dude, no problem! There are plenty of other men out there!

On our second date, I unabashedly admitted sitting in my own vulnerability, "I have herpes. I don't know if it's going to change the way you feel about dating me, but I just want to be very honest before we go further." He replied without hesitation, "Don't a whole bunch of people have it? It's pretty prevalent, right? Does it really matter? Do you have an outbreak right now? No? Okay, I say, Let's Go For It!"

I held my breath after the weekend ended to see how Dan would process our time together and my admission. Would he change his mind when he had time alone? I held my breath when I received a text from him the following Monday morning:

11/17/15, 9:41 AM

Morning sweets! I'm super busy today but wanted to send you a big kiss and tell you I thought about our wonderful Saturday and Sunday

▬▬▬▬ I didn't think a woman like you was out there but there you are 😊

FROM THE OTHER SIDE OF THE LOOKING GLASS

"Often, it's not about becoming a new person, but becoming the person you were meant to be, and already are, but don't know how to be."

— Heath L. Buckmaster, Box of Hair: A Fairy Tale

Guys can take care of themselves; they are big boys. It is not for me to manage a guys' reaction. Once I choose to give them full disclosure, their reaction is up to them. Two powerful people choosing to coalesce together make a much stronger couple.

You may not admit to having herpes perfectly the first time. As you can see from my stories, I did not say or act perfectly. I realize that I could not be expected to do it perfectly the first time. I had to practice. Luckily, I was dating so I was in a situation where there were practice opportunities. From these experiences, I learned exactly what I was supposed to learn - to gain comfort speaking about herpes and realize how to grow from making mistakes! Perhaps my lesson was to learn from the conversation, make an adjustment, and do it again. The more and more I honed how to tell my partner, the more I attracted a very different quality of man and partner. By identifying with herpes proudly, I drew men that were open, mature, and aware.

Having herpes is a natural filter for partners. I did not know I had a sifter existing in my back pocket. I was making choices with men previously based on the assumption that I was damaged goods and not worthy of the purest form of love. By not being in love with myself, I was attracting men who did not love themselves or were not fully awakened in all aspects of their lives. Naively, I felt when a relationship did not work out, I was responsible for its deterioration. I obsessed over what I could have done differently, when, in reality, it was a mismatch. The universe was redirecting opportunities to find partners better aligned with me. My once viewed "dating failures" were, in fact, positive feedback preparing me for the next powerful life changing partner. I was refining my own process without realizing it. What a beautiful and blissful process when I look back at it!

Love, Safety, and Belonging are three vital needs. Maslow's Hierarchy of Basic Needs brings to light essential relationship needs once physical survival and safety needs are met. Maslow states: "The person… will hunger for affectionate relationships with people in general for a place in the group."

In past relationships, I expended so much energy trying to look and act like the perfect package and partner, treating them well, doing extra work, and managing many workarounds to meet their needs. Inadvertently, they became more important than attention on myself. I believed that by offering them my family, acceptance, love, finances, and intimacy, my partners would, in turn, offer it back to me. Subconsciously, I was seeking a man to complete and fulfill me, instead of investing in myself to embody this core value and foundational need. This violation denied my own powerful essence and, once corrected, the universe tidied the mixed signals and abundantly provided happiness multifold. I want you, my reader, to know that you are significant, that your true self matters.

It takes time to accept the diagnosis of herpes.
- **For you, the patient:** give yourself time to process and grieve, I realize you are out of our comfort zone. Elisabeth Kübler-Ross is a psychiatrist whose groundbreaking book *On Death and Dying* in 1969 postulates a series of emotions experienced by survivors after an intimate's death. The 5 Stages of Grieving are denial, anger, bargaining, depression, and acceptance.

  The diagnosis of herpes is a dramatic, life-changing event where this grieving process can also occur. I encourage being conscious of this transition, which will not happen overnight. Herpes can be a curse threatening to upend us, or it can be a slingshot into new emotional growth. Sometimes we suppress and shy away from things that can be dangerous, but advantageously, the momentum can propel you forward into a better life. The events we overcome become monumental parts of who we are; let us use this tool to expand our world.

- **For your partner:** give them time to digest. Herpes does affect someone's life, and I have discovered if that person does not like it, this has nothing to do with my self-worth and self-love. This person does not like the virus and/or the concept of it. In time, you will develop the mental toughness and strategies to cope with moving on, coupled with a strong sense of self-worth, the experience will be one to build on.

There is power in letting an experience change us. Acquiring herpes may have been given to you out of your control. Perhaps you gave it to others. Regardless, we can choose to grow from it, rather than crumble under the experience. There is power in telling others the truth. There is power in having choices. In the end, feeling powerful, women can be exponentially incredible. The more I embraced and identified with herpes, the more awakened my world became and multiple opportunities came forward, particularly in the world of dating.

It takes work to get what you want. I would have loved for all of this to have been figured out for me without having to lift a finger or my voice. My initial goal working with Julien was to be able to look back in my mid-50s and feel independent, emotionally strong, secure, and loved if children or marriage was not in my future. Being honest about herpes was the release I was looking for. Having herpes or any other ailment is not about being in resistance to yourself in terms of denying, blaming, shaming, pointing fingers; it is about perspective and wanting things badly enough to tell the truth. For me, it was wanting a healthy relationship with an equal partner.

> *"Let us think of education as the means of developing our greatest abilities, because in each of us there is a private hope and dream which, fulfilled, can be translated into benefit for everyone and greater strength for our nation."*
>
> — John F. Kennedy

Pay It Forward is an expression for describing when the recipient of a good deed repays it to others, instead of the original donator. Julien did this for me, and in turn, I give this gift to my patients in the office and to you, my reader. Spread this information like wildfire! I believe my patients have benefited from my compassion and wealth of experiences in this regard. Let us create a positive community of education, responsibility, and strength surrounding herpes.

Chapter Two

DR. LOANZON VERSUS SHEILA LOANZON

"To err is human; to forgive, divine."
— Alexander Pope An Essay on Criticism, Part II, 1711.

THE ABOVE PROVERB expresses the idea that forgiveness is a worthy response to human failings, as anyone can make a mistake. This proverb is often quoted in response to preventable medical errors. It also appropriately addresses the tension of how I acted as a physician as opposed to how I behaved in my personal life. Physicians often joke that we make the worst patients, usually when we miss our own doctors' appointments, fail to keep up our exercise regimes, or forget to take prescribed medications. At the same time, we expend tremendous amounts of energy keeping patients alive and safe.

While a multitude of patients have their opinion regarding their personal physician or interaction with other physicians, my experience over nine years in ob-gyn residency and as an attending has brought me joy and fulfillment every day. I would like to reassure the readers and my patients of my unending devotion to you and your health. The painstaking hours poring over medical journals, memorizing and learning, sacrificing time away from family and friends, running around the hospital saving mothers and their baby's lives, toiling away extensively during surgery dissecting and controlling a small bleeding pedicle has been worth it. Through my high scores in patient satisfaction assessments, patients seem to have reassuring interactions with me after an office visit, delivery, or surgery. I absolutely enjoy my chosen profession; my patients bring delight and daily challenges in abundance, which I meet with ease and attentiveness. I truly believe I am doing exactly what I am supposed to do in this world in terms of my career.

Reflecting back on myself as a 23-year-old first-year medical school student, I stood proudly wearing my white coat for the first time and, in front of family, ceremoniously recited the Osteopathic Oath, the Osteopathic version of the Hippocratic Oath.

The Osteopathic Oath

I do hereby affirm my loyalty to the profession I am about to enter.

I will be mindful always of my great responsibility to preserve the health and the life of my patients, to retain their respect both as a physician and a friend who will guard their secrets with scrupulous honor and fidelity, to perform faithfully my professional duties, to employ only those recognized methods of treatment consistent with good judgement and with my skill and ability, keeping in mind always nature's laws and the body's inherent capacity for recovery.

I will be ever vigilant in aiding in the general welfare of the community, sustaining its laws and institutions, not engaging in those practices which will in any way bring shame or discredit upon myself or my profession. I will give no drugs for deadly purposes to any person, though it be asked of me.

I will endeavor to work in accord with my colleagues in a spirit of progressive cooperation, and never by work or by act cast imputations upon them or their rightful practices.

I will look with respect and esteem upon all those who have taught me my art. To my college I will be loyal and strive always for its best interests and for the interests of the students who will come after me. I will be ever alert to further the application of basic biologic truths to the healing arts and to develop the principles of osteopathy.

This version of the Osteopathic Oath has been in use since 1954. The Hippocratic Oath is one of the oldest binding documents in history. Written in antiquity, its principles are held sacred by doctors to this day: treat the sick to the best of one's ability, preserve patient privacy, teach the secrets of medicine to the next generation, and so on. The American Medical Association's Oath of Hippocrates (1996 edition) "has remained in Western civilization as an expression of ideal conduct for the physician." Today, most graduating medical school students swear to some form of the oath, usually a modernized version adapted to current social views.

The instant high regard and mystique that comes with the noble medical profession is gratifying and awe-inspiring. As I worked my way through medical school, I had my eye on the prize ... get that degree! I did not allow myself to understand the magnitude of the goal that I was striving for; I was focused on passing class after class, anatomy labs after clinical skill days. The family events that I was missing, the social events that my friends outside medicine were attending, the lack of sleep I was accruing: all of this was a small sacrifice for my dreams. At 27 years old, I stood at graduation on top of my educational mountain as Dr. Loanzon, and the sense of pride and accomplishment was rightfully earned.

Physician Persona

There are several key personality adjustments acquired in medical school to survive. This is not written formally into medical textbooks, but absorbed through my studies of my profession. In medicine, there is a favorite teaching phrase: "See one, Do one, Teach one." It generally relates to a procedure taught to a junior physician that means observe a procedure once, perform the procedure under guidance once, and then teach others the same procedure indefinitely. This concept also applies to various aspects of the social realm of being a doctor.

My physician persona was created as most people assume different school, work, home, and social group personalities. I remember standing at that White Coat Ceremony, observing older teaching physicians walk through the auditorium with an air of pride and confidence that would cause a patient to give them instant respect. My mama would point them out, beaming and whispering, "Look at that distinguished physician over there. And over there, too. You are going to be just like them!" *I* was joining this elite group?!?! What a privilege!

From that White Coat ceremony on, I tried so hard to be perfect, intelligent, caring, and important, as I believed a respectable doctor should be. In medical school, I began to embody this image of a future doctor and imposed it on to others around me. Rest assured, my medical school buddies were attempting to find their own distinguished persona to survive the world of being a health care provider, as well. The need to be accepted and fit in was important to me, and I created a personal dream of what I would look like for my own self in this field as a doctor.

As a physician, I mastered that personality well and the image for certain circumstances, too. It is not uncommon that as an intern I pretended and projected a certain image to get through a hospital call, surgery, and interactions with patients. A great friend of mine who attended a different medical school at the same time joked, "Sheila, we have to fake it 'til we make it!"

Professional Detachment

Early on in medical school, I also learned of "professional detachment." It is an unnatural skill used to traverse through one's career in medicine and ultimately help patients. As cold as it sounds, I learned to suppress my innate sympathy to function in the medical environment. This facilitated the capability for me to care for multiple complex patients and complete my job to the best of my ability. The patient becomes reduced to medical facts of the case; emotions can complicate crucial decisions about patients' care. Psychological stress can be minimized by maintaining a distance but, more important, patients safely stay alive. The benefit is positive in favor of the patient and the clinician. I avoid letting my personal beliefs or biases cloud medical conclusions, and I also avoid bringing emotionally draining work into my personal life. I had one physician during residency succinctly advise me after I had spent hours with a patient at bedside who was diagnosed with cancer, "Young Doctor Loanzon, the *patient* is the one with the disease."

I did not realize that I disconnected within the first few weeks of school when it came to the textbook medicine. Studying microbiology, it was not a real clinical diagnosis to me, just "bugs on a paper" to memorize to pass the next exam. I discussed herpes and other viruses readily with my study group at Starbucks over caffeine-charged drinks, but did not connect that we were reviewing and perfecting our knowledge of a sexually transmitted infection that I housed in my body.

Doctors Practice Medicine; Doctors are Human, Too

So now, after medical school graduation, stood this bold doctor persona with all the knowledge of medicine but disjointed from the subject matter. For many years, I scooted along in this world as Dr. Loanzon, the confident, esteemed surgeon in the office and hospital during the day, and grappled with Sheila, the timid, insecure, and shy girl of my 20s and early 30s, during my off hours.

It was only until I worked with Julien that I realized the tension of acting as a doctor and behaving as a patient did not coexist well within me. Pride got the best of me, and then it seemed too hard to right my wrongs. The desire to look perfect in medicine was too great and to admit to herpes without self-confidence and self-love to support me seemed unattainable. Referring back to my professional oath, was I performing to my "ideal conduct?" If I admit this, would I look stupid and renounce my professional doctrine? Could I own the persona of being the doctor who has herpes but could not protect herself from it? Can I admit to being a doctor who was diagnosed and did not know how to verbalize it to her partners but could rattle off facts to her patients?

I spend my time healing people, serving humanity, and improving quality of life for my patients, yet the fulfillment in my personal life suffered until now. The disparity between following a creed professionally and not following a similar doctrine personally created mental and emotional turmoil for me, consciously and subconsciously. The seams of these two personalities no longer seemed smooth. Acknowledging that I have herpes has been a challenge. By being a great doctor, I was informing and educating patients about how to treat outbreaks, engage in safe sexual activity, and live and thrive with the virus. Ironically, I was not acting as a great patient and absorbing the gravity of my diagnosis. I believed there could only be punishment, suffering, and judgment for me, an attitude I worked to prevent with my patients through open, trusting dialogue, and education. The strength taken to consciously choose to stop feeling guilty and punish myself and instead move forward and change my ingrained attitude patterns has been challenging but eventually rewarding.

I realize it is acceptable to have these two perspectives. It is natural and understandable. My efforts to marry my personal and professional life have not been easy; however, I continuously strive to combine these worlds. I am not proud of hiding herpes from my partners, and I do not intend to diminish my poor and inappropriate actions of the past. I forgive myself; at the time, my actions were necessary for my survival. I accept this was my survival strategy. These two parts of myself were to be in sync for me to expand myself—not only as a doctor, but also as an integral human being improving my own quality of life. What I came to realize is that I wanted to take my oath from being a professional commitment into a personal one. I now hold myself to the same standards personally as I do professionally.

This book is my personal commitment and step in combining both parts of myself into one. The compassion I have felt during coaching is one that I extend to you. If you fall, I can give you my hand. I can help you stand up while saying, "You can do it; go ahead."

Chapter Three

WHEN IT COMES TO HERPES DON'T BELIEVE THE INTERNET - ALSO KNOWN AS COMMON MYTHS

"The fewer the facts, the stronger the opinion."

— Arnold H. Glasow

WHENEVER AN OBSTETRIC or gynecologic patient comes to see me in the office, I inevitably end up encouraging them, "Please don't Google. If you have any questions, talk to me." This usually is met with a chuckle and admittance that they already have. I appreciate the subsequent emails requesting information from my knowledge and perspective. This generally comes from a space of being overwhelmed with the large amount of knowledge on the Internet, difficulty in knowing what is true or not, and also strong desire for pertinent information from a professional they trust. Here are some of the existing myths that need to be dispelled. The following chapter reviews the facts.

Myth: Only Promiscuous, Dirty People Get Herpes.

A standardized false concept pertaining to herpes is the notion that a person must have slept with multiple people to acquire the infection.

Education: It only takes *one* sexual act with *one* herpes positive person to be exposed to the virus.

Myth: You Can Get Genital Herpes From the Toilet Seat and Other Inanimate Objects.

Clinical scenario: A patient came to see me when she had a vaginal ulcer. She believed she received herpes from a toilet seat when water splashed her when she was flushing. Upon examination, she in fact had fissures from a yeast infection from uncontrolled diabetic blood sugars.

Clinical scenario: A patient who married her high school sweetheart came to me for STD testing. Her husband, a police officer, whom were each other's first sexual partners, tested positive for chlamydia and herpes. She recounts his story, "He went to a house call for disturbance of the peace. A woman threw a towel at his pants while she was trying to run away, and he says he must have gotten it that way. Is that possible, or am I being naive?" Reiterating the sexual nature in which sexually transmitted conditions are spread, she sheepishly realized her husband had an extramarital affair.

Clinical scenario: When Danielle, a herpes positive patient, first started dating her fiancé, David, he was allergic to latex and had very sensitive skin. He used polypropylene condoms for safe sex. One day he noticed a tender rash at the base of his penis and got it checked out. He was shocked to be told it was herpes because he always wore condoms. David was very ashamed that he was "unclean" and so fearful that he would give herpes to his children that he stopped swimming in the family pool and would not let the children use the same shower he had used.

Education: Herpes enters into the human body through inoculations of mucous membranes by touching, kissing, and sexual vaginal, anal, and oral sex. These membranes are moist linings of orifices and internal parts of the body, including the eyes, mouth, vulva, vagina, and rectum, amongst other organs. A break in the skin can allow entry, so it is important to wash hands so that fluid from the herpes vesicle does not spread to other parts of your body or to others.

It is not possible to obtain herpes from a towel in a hotel room or from gym equipment. A person cannot get herpes by sharing meals, drinks, or straws. It is a good rule of thumb not to use anyone else's lipstick, toothbrush, and lip balm. If you have chapped lips or break in the skin and swipe on a lipstick that someone with herpes used (with or without a visible oral outbreak), then you are more susceptible to contracting herpes. It is most likely low risk, but there is still a small degree of risk.

If using sex toys, it is important to wash the toy before and after use and do not share. Spreading the virus could occur if a sex toy is taken from one partner and immediately used on another partner, as the vesicular fluid may be present.

Triggers can exist, causing patients to have herpes episodes, notably stress, waxing or shaving pubic hair, or onset of menses.

Myth: Blood Tests Confirm Herpes

Patients asking for an STI screening from their physician expect herpes to be included in the STI panel. Blood testing for the presence of herpes has fallen out of favor as a routine test as it is non-specific. A culture of a lesion is the gold standard of evaluation. Blood tests are often expensive and falsely positive. As a clinician, it is important to have the correct positive diagnosis from an outbreak lesion before delivering a diagnosis due to the adverse psychological effects it can incur.

Clinical scenario: Patient via secure email messaging: "I would like complete STD screening. I don't have any symptoms but would like to have a clean bill of health for peace of mind."

Clinician: "No problem. I have ordered urine and blood testing. Please go to the lab and complete at your convenience."

Urine STI screening is checking for gonorrhea and chlamydia; serum (blood) testing is checking for HIV, syphilis, Hepatitis B and sometimes Hepatitis C. A cervical swab obtained in the office can also check for gonorrhea and chlamydia. Patients assume herpes is included in blood testing but usually it is not.

Education: The Centers for Disease Control and Prevention[2] (CDC) does not recommend routine testing for herpes because STI screening is done for infections that have serious outcomes if left untreated. Gonorrhea and chlamydia can cause infertility. Syphilis can cause neurological symptoms. Hepatitis B and C can cause liver issues, and HIV causes multiple issues with multi-organ involvement.

Herpes is treated successfully with antiviral medications and, while it may have lifestyle implications, does not cause untreatable infections or have the same impact on a population as other infections. The CDC does not currently recommend routine herpes testing in patients without symptoms (i.e., outbreaks) suggestive of the infection. It is not clear that identification of people with herpes will actually decrease the spread of the virus within the population.

---

[2] The Centers for Disease Control and Prevention (CDC) is the leading national public health institute of the United States. The CDC is a federal agency under the Department of Health and Human Services and is head-quartered in Georgia.

Its main goal is to protect public health and safety through the control and prevention of disease, injury, and disability. The CDC focuses national attention on developing and applying disease control and prevention. It especially focuses its attention on infectious disease, food borne pathogens, environmental health, occupational safety and health, health promotion, injury prevention, and educational activities designed to improve the health of United States citizens. In addition, the CDC researches and provides information on non-infectious diseases such as obesity and diabetes.

Research shows that detection of herpes does not necessarily lead to changes in sexual behavior, so at this point, routine screening of asymptomatic people is not recommended.

Myth: An Ulceration on My Rectum is Not Herpes.

Genital herpes can present at any mucus membranes such as the perineum, vulva, rectum, and anus area. Some patients can begin their herpes history with sores on their vagina and throughout life only get outbreaks on the rectum. Skin fissures can be a herpes outbreak, and a culture can help confirm if the herpes virus is present or not. It is important to note that women can get fissures or ulcers from yeast infections, syphilis, hemorrhoids, ingrown hairs from waxing or shaving, pimples, Behcet's ulcers, inflammatory bowel disease, and aphthous ulcers (canker sores). Many lesions in the genital area can present with sores, and it is best to not Google (it might freak you out!) and to see your healthcare provider for confirmation on your diagnosis.

Myth: I was just diagnosed with herpes, so it must have come from my current partner.

Herpes can lay dormant and is not always expressed immediately. Therefore, this may be the first recognized outbreak; it does not necessarily mean that this is your first exposure. We cannot know if it came from this partner or your first partner.

Myth: I don't have medical insurance, so I can't be tested.

While I work for an organization where lab testing is prevalent, government-funded clinics exist and testing can be done through them. Most counties have public health departments that offer low or no-cost STI screening. Planned Parenthood is also an excellent resource for STI testing and contraception if you do not have insurance or need medical services on a sliding-fee scale.

HOW TO AVOID COMMON MISTAKES WOMEN MAKE

Talk to your partner before getting busy!

Sexual intimacy can be very exciting, while conversational intimacy can be extremely difficult. As empowered and open with our bodies as women can be, we are in a different culture than our parents characterized by internet dating, stable careers with financial independence, and women getting married at older ages. It is important for you both to share your STI histories. It can be a difficult conversation, and while fear of judgment or ruining the moment is present, it is the responsible thing to do. Certainly use of condoms can help protect you if you decide not to have the conversation. I understand the hype and excitement of being in the moment; however, thinking, "we will figure out whatever results come of this," may not always be in your best health interest.

Open your eyes and see what is in front of you!

I know it seems very awkward, but it is best to look at your partner before becoming intimate. Women feel it is impolite to stare, but you may not realize that there is an outbreak or genital wart. Men are not always upfront with their history, aware of their bodies, or go to their physicians as regularly as women see their gynecologist. While there may not be an outbreak present to view, it is the responsible thing to do.

Grab a mirror and get to know yourself!

Just as much as women check their face, teeth, or hair, I recommend that women also check their genitalia. It is skin that can become cancerous and abnormal, and it is an important part of hygiene and self-care. Evaluating your skin and anatomy provides a baseline if something changes in the future. Just as we recommend breast exams and mole checks, getting to know when your body is normal and abnormal are important.

I appreciate that you might NOT want to come in and see me; however, it is a good idea!

Patients run the gamut on this: some women come in too frequently; others do not come in soon enough. The thought process usually looks like: "I thought that I would wait." "I wanted to keep waiting." "I wasn't really quite sure and thought it would go away," "I put Neosporin/Vaseline/ice on it, and it seemed to get better," "Google said it would be okay." Usually after a time of minimal improvement, they arrive in the office. At that time, it may be too late to do the culture and get a positive result.

Ideally, it is best to diagnose herpes at the first sign that a lesion is present. This culture will give us the definitive diagnosis. The test has poor accuracy once the lesions are crusted over, and it becomes a clinical judgment of your health care provider looking at the lesions. If we miss that window of diagnosis, we can simply repeat it the next time an outbreak occurs and go from there.

I don't have vaginal sex. I am 100% safe from getting herpes and any other STDs.

The only way to avoid STIs is abstaining from vaginal, oral, or anal sex. By using condoms 100% of the time and being in a long-term, mutually monogamous relationship, the chance of herpes is lowered. It is possible to have more than one STI at a time, for example, herpes and chlamydia. Therefore, I recommend both partners be tested and have negative results prior to sexual interaction.

However, it is important to understand that condoms may not always fully protect against herpes. Herpes can occur in both men and women's genital areas that are covered by latex condoms, but can also occur in any area that is not fully covered by the condom, such as mouth, tongue, anus, rectum, perineum, and testicles. Many people have herpes simplex viruses but may not know it because they are asymptomatic. Even if they have never had symptoms, they could still pass it to you.

I am scared to get an STD test. I would rather just not know.

Some women are afraid of getting STI testing. If you are making a mature choice to be sexually active, please be mature enough to face the realities of STI screening. Sexually transmitted infections exist and treatment is available.

Clinical scenario: Anna, a 28-year-old patient who is dating an older gentleman, comes to me for abnormal pap smears. Every year I see her and she asks me for STI testing. Three years later, she is still working up the courage to complete the screening. She is plagued with the push/pull of wanting to make sure she is clear of infection and feeling trepidation if knowing is better than not knowing. Anna feels that her abnormal pap smear is bad enough, and she is not sure she can handle any more "bad" news. The ramifications of a positive test are too great for her because it brings up other issues: what does this mean about her partner? What does this mean for her relationship? Can she trust again? I respect her protective mechanism stance as her adult choice; however, obtaining knowledge and reassurance seems greater than being uninformed.

Chapter Four

GENITAL HERPES: STIGMA STILL STRONG

What percentage of the population actually carries the virus, and what does this mean?

ACCORDING TO the CDC in 2016[3], in people aged 14-49, one in six has genital herpes. This means 16.7% of the population has the virus.

There are several interesting facts in our current world that has the same ratio of one in six.

- One in six people in America face hunger.
- In 2010, NBC News claimed one in six students are regularly bullied.
- Various data state one in six people might have Irritable Bowel Syndrome.
- One in six men have experienced abusive sexual experiences before age 18.
- One in six American women have been victims of attempted or completed rape in their lifetime.
- Approximately one in seven men are diagnosed with prostate cancer during their lifetime.

---

[3] Reference: "Genital Herpes - STD Information from CDC." 2016. Accessed April 11. http://www.cdc.gov/std/herpes/default.htm.

Television commercials regularly display information and support groups for hunger, bullying, and Irritable Bowel Syndrome, but public knowledge of herpes is limited. I encourage you to calculate how many people you know who have irritable bowel syndrome—one in six of those people also could have herpes.

According to the CDC in 2014, one in 11 people had Diabetes Mellitus in the United States. If we think about family members, friends, and coworkers we know who have diabetes, there are more people who have herpes than diabetes! Diabetes is so prevalent and accepted, yet herpes has sexual stigma. We have an opportunity to educate and open knowledge about this topic, and I would like to start here.

What are the stigmas around herpes and where do they come from?

Popular stigmas include people assuming that someone who has herpes is dirty and that the person must have been sexually involved with multiple people. Fear of contracting herpes plays a role. Due to lack of knowledge, the awareness of contracting herpes is heightened. Therefore, all items touched by someone with herpes are a contagious item, which is absolutely not true. Oftentimes, I find patients are judgmental of themselves and are concerned that friends will avoid and judge them, too. Also, if a diagnosis comes from an untoward situation like infidelity, herpes also carries that negativity.

It is very common for physicians to have difficulty speaking about it. I would like to believe that we physicians are in the role of being open and honest with patients and do what is right; however, some health care providers may not feel comfortable. So when you, the patient, come to us for advice and knowledge and the physician does not feel comfortable discussing the topic and/or has their own judgements, the stigma is perpetuated.

How does pop culture portray herpes?

On *Saturday Night Live* in 2006, Amy Poehler played the clueless housewife in a facetious Valtrex commercial where she contracts herpes from her supposedly faithful husband, played by Alec Baldwin. In a 2014 episode of *Inside Amy Schumer*, Amy tries to negotiate with God to protect her from getting herpes. God, played by Paul Giamatti, retorts, "70 percent of people who reach out to me are having a herpes scare." In our culture due to the stigma of herpes, jokes are made and we all continue to laugh and thus the jokes continue. It is difficult to stop the jokes and educate in a social situation.

Did pharmaceutical companies create the herpes stigma for profit?[4] Did *Time* magazine ruin herpes for our generation?[5]

In 1982, all eyes were on the herpes simplex. In the previous two decades, the public perception of the benign-but-irritating virus had transformed from "it itches down there" into the scourge of a generation. That year, *Time* magazine ran a cover story titled "The New Scarlet Letter", which explored---and reinforced—the stigma surrounding herpes. The authors, John Leo and Maureen Dowd, argue that herpes could put an end to the so-called sexual revolution, which they clearly disdained. (In fact, the opening sentence of the feature reads, "After chastity slouched off into exile in the '60's, the sexual revolution encountered little resistance.")

The story declared herpes to be "altering sexual rites in America, changing courtship patterns, sending thousands of

---

[4] https://broadly.vice.com/en_us/article/did-big-pharma-create-the-herpes-stigma-for-profit

[5] https://ellacydawson.wordpress.com/2015/07/25/time-magazine-ruined-herpes-journalism-heres-how-to-fix-it

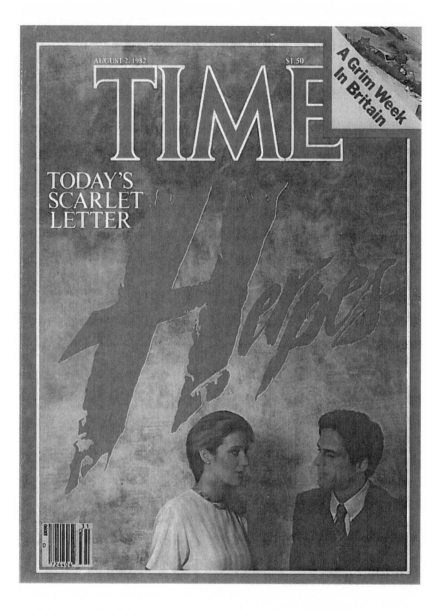

sufferers spinning into months of depression and self-exile and delivering a numbing blow to the one-night stand." It emphasized the authors' expectation that "the herpes counter revolution may be ushering a reluctant, grudging chastity back into fashion." Herpes is portrayed as a scourge of swingers, prostitutes, and philanderers. Women quoted in the article "give husbands smiling lectures on the ravages of the disease to keep them faithful." In the course of the piece, there are references to the Age of Guilt and the "VD of the Ivy League." The authors conclude their article by thanking herpes for "helping to bring to a close an era of mindless promiscuity" and "ushering in a period in which sex is linked more firmly to commitment and trust."

Although the *Time* story is reduced to irresponsible journalism by Leo and Dowd, the narratives outlined are still portrayed in the media and remnants of this thought process present today. Jenelle Marie Davis, founder of the award-winning STD Project and a spokesperson for PositiveSingles.com (a dating site for people with STDs), provides resources to thousands of women and men facing the same social backlash, stigma, and shame as when she was diagnosed at 16 years old. Davis states, "When there's been research done about what the consequences of herpes are and what people are most afraid of, it's the social ramifications. Most people don't care about the virus itself: They care about how the virus is perceived."

Davis has also said, "People get infections all the time—viral colds and flu—and no one shames those people because there is no 'you did something bad to get this.' As a society, we tell people how and who to have sex with, then you add a taboo infection as a result of being sexually active, and people go crazy."

According to a study published in *The New England Journal of Medicine*, "For many patients, the psychological effects are far more severe than the physical consequences of the disease. Shock, anger, guilt, low self-esteem, fear of transmitting the infection to others, and impaired sexual function are common and can interfere substantially with relationships." Herpes diagnosis can also lead to social withdrawal and isolation, particularly in young people.

Studies show that many doctors overlook the psychological toll herpes can take and focus exclusively on treatment of physical symptoms. A few conspiring circumstances surround the stigmatization of herpes, which began sometime in the 1970s. Up until the 1960s, doctors were not able to distinguish between HSV 1 (better known as oral herpes or cold sores) and HSV 2 (characterized frequently by genital sores). Cold sores on your mouth or genitals were all considered herpes. Then the differentiation between HSV 1 and HSV 2 occurred, and immediately there was a "good" and "bad" virus. Herpes on your mouth indicated appropriate behavior, but genital herpes becomes a moral sexual issue.

There are many unproven, yet fascinating, rumors that blame Burroughs Wellcome Co., the pharmaceutical company behind the antiviral medication Acyclovir, for developing the herpes stigma in tandem with their new drug in order to create a market for it. In the late 1970s, a disease-awareness campaign was organized to alert doctors and patients to the benefits of the new drug. In America, Burroughs Wellcome sponsored support groups to advise "sufferers" of the benefits of the new drug. Pedro Cuatrecasas, a biochemist who was involved in the discovery, development, and marketing of Acyclovir as the head of Research & Design from 1975 to 1985 recalls: "During the [discovery and development] of Acyclovir, marketing insisted that there were 'no markets' for this compound. Most had hardly heard of genital herpes, to say nothing about the common and devastating system herpetic infections in immunocompromised patients." By 1983, an article featuring pharmaceutical analyst Arnold Snider told *The New York Times*, "My guess would be that most pharmaceutical companies have a program for genital herpes. It is quite an enormous effort right now." The *Times* concluded, "The current herpes epidemic presents a rare opportunity in the drug business—a potentially booming new market with potentially booming profits."

Taboo STD Topics

Harris Interactive conducted a poll between December 14, 2006 and January 12, 2007 commissioned by the drug company Novartis.[6] The poll included 503 US adults with genital herpes and ~1400 other adults who said they did not have genital herpes. Participants answered questions about their relationships, social stigmas, and views of potentially taboo topics, including HIV, genital herpes, mental illness, obesity, substance abuse, and cancer.

64% of participants without genital herpes and 56% of herpes positive participants did not think any of those topics were taboo. Social stigma was evaluated, and out of all the sexually transmitted diseases, HIV ranked first and genital herpes ranked second.

Among genital herpes patients, 39% were troubled by societal stigma about genital herpes. Far more genital herpes patients (75%) were troubled by bothersome symptoms of genital herpes outbreaks. Among people with genital herpes, 36% said they tell their partners about their genital herpes "well in advance of having sexual intercourse for the first time" and 68% were concerned about transmitting genital herpes to their sexual partners.

This poll also found that this does not mean that it is easy for patients to talk to their partners about genital herpes. For instance, in 325 genital herpes patients who reported having genital herpes outbreaks, 38% said they made up an excuse to

6 Reference: http://www.cbsnews.com/news/genital-herpes-stigma-still-strong/ by Miranda Hitti, Reviewed by Louise Chang, B) 2005-2006 WebMD, Inc. All rights reserved, Copyright 2007 WebMD, LLC. All Rights Reserved.

avoid having sex during an outbreak, instead of telling their partner about their outbreak.

Most people without genital herpes said they would avoid having a relationship with someone who has genital herpes and would break up with a partner who had genital herpes.

This stigma is perpetuated by lack of knowledge, pop culture, and its sexual acquisition. I would like to create a movement of positivity, understanding, and awareness. When people have that, the stigma will change. Through educating the public, we can change the perspective and eradicate the stigma.

There can often be anger that is directed at the current partner, and fidelity is often questioned in those cases. It is important to realize that even though someone has a first diagnosed outbreak, it does not necessarily mean this is a new exposure.

A COMMON SECRET: COMMUNITIES FIGHTING TOGETHER TO BATTLE THE STIGMA OF HERPES

What are other people doing to dispel myths and educate - activists, celebrities?

Celebrities often use their fame to help raise awareness for diseases and health related causes. However, no celebrity has come forward claiming herpes. Due to the stigma of the virus, there are only speculations of celebrities who have herpes and this is based off of oral outbreaks captured on camera by the media. Online lists exist for possible celebrities and athletes who have been prescribed antiviral medication however the majority of STD lists focus on those celebrity figures who have HIV and Hepatitis C. The only time we hear a celebrity has genital herpes is in the context of a scandalous rumor, bitter divorce, or lawsuit.[7]

---

[7] http://www.thestdproject.com/stigma-genital-herpes-and-stds/

There are several pioneers who have stepped forward to create a movement in normalizing herpes in modern society. A young activist named Ella Dawson, a 21-year-old college student from the UK, is advocating to remove the stigma of herpes. She has a popular blog at https://ellacydawson.wordpress.com/, where she increases herpes awareness and education. She is also featured in TEDx talks where she claims: "STIs aren't a consequence. They are inevitable." She has said in interviews, "When a real person—a woman you know and respect—casually mentions having herpes, it stops being a punch line and starts being someone's reality."

Adriel Dale[8], a 36 year old who was diagnosed with HSV 2 in 2005, was terrified about having to reveal a secret that had brought him to shame for years. He noticed a pattern and judged his herpes diagnosis as a sentence to his love life. Today, Dale is a life coach and the founder of Herpes Opportunity, which helps people cope with herpes through blog posts, forums, and weekend retreats that bring herpes positive people together. Dale concedes that accepting his diagnosis was not easy and what helped was having a support group. Also realizing that herpes infections are common and can happen to anyone. "The more we shame and judge those 'dirty people with herpes,' the more ashamed they are of disclosing and saying that, yeah, it's just a skin condition," Dale said.

---

[8] Adriel Dale is a life coach and the founder of Herpes Opportunity, helping people cope with herpes through blog posts, forums and weekend retreats that bring herpes-positive people together. http://www.npr.org/sections/health-shots/2016/01/22/463845334/a-common-secret-struggling-with-the-stigma-of-herpes

Chapter Five

JUST THE FACTS - HERPES 101

"Facts do not cease to exist because they are ignored."

— Aldous Huxley, *Complete Essays 2*, 1926–29

I HAVE INCLUDED in this book the most poignant facts and points for the target audience reading the book. New literature and studies constantly come out with multiple aspects of the discussion. This book is not all encompassing, but I found the best take-home messages that resonated with myself, and with patients. Nuances exist with herpes, and there is a multitude of medical information that I have abbreviated here. This does not diminish information out there, and I encourage contact with a health care provider if you have further questions.

You may have noted in this book that I have repeated several concepts. This tactic is not meant to be repetitive but to highlight what you may pick up at different times of this book. 40–80% of medical information provided by healthcare practitioners is forgotten immediately. The greater the amount of information presented, the lower the proportion correctly recalled[9]. Furthermore, almost half of the information that is remembered is incorrect[10]. Luckily, you have this book to refer back to!

---

[9] McGuire LC. Remembering what the doctor said: organization and older adults' memory for medical information. Exp Aging Res 1996; 22:403–28.

[10] Anderson JL, Dodman S, Kopelman M, Fleming A. Patient information recall in a rheumatology clinic. Rheumatol Rehabil 1979; 18:245–55.

What are the types of herpes, and what are their differences and similarities?

Genital herpes is a sexually transmitted disease. There are two types of herpes viruses: Herpes Simplex Type 1 (HSV 1) and Herpes Simplex Type 2 (HSV 2). When an exposure occurs, the herpes vesicle carries the virus. Contact with this fluid causes infection. Herpes can be contracted from an infected sex partner who does not have a visible sore or even know that they are carrying the virus. The virus is released to the skin and then spread to the partner. Because patients can be asymptomatic and spread the virus, this is how the infection exposure is so rampant.

Historically, HSV 1 indicated oral herpes outbreaks versus HSV 2 represented genital outbreaks. However due to the prevalence of oral sex, HSV 1 can be found on positive genital cultures. HSV 1 has increased in frequency and is estimated to be responsible for new herpes genital infections in the United States[11].

In the US, approximately 50 million people are infected with HSV 2. Genital herpes is frequently under recognized because the infection is often subclinical. For instance, in a population-based cross-sectional survey of adults living in New York City in 2004, nearly 28% were infected with herpes and 88% had no prior knowledge of their diagnosis[12]. A prior infection of HSV 1

---

[11] Bernstein DI, Bellamy AR, Hook EW 3rd, Levin MJ, Wald A, Ewell MG, Wolff PA, Deal CD, Heineman TC, Dubin G, Belshe RB. Epidemiology, clinical presentation, and antibody response to primary infection with herpes simplex virus type 1 and type 2 in young women. Clin Infect Dis. 2013 Feb; 56(3):344–51. Epub 2012 Nov 29.
[12] Langenberg AG, Corey L, Ashley RL, et al. A prospective study of new infections with herpes simplex virus type 1 and type 2. Chiron HSV Vaccine Study Group. N Engl J Med 1999; 341:1432.
Schillinger JA, McKinney CM, Garg R, et al. Seroprevalence of herpes simplex virus type 2 and characteristics associated with undiagnosed infection:New York City, 2004. Sex Transm Dis 2008; 35:599.
Gupta R, Warren T, Wald A. Genital herpes.Lancet. 2007; 370(9605):2127.

also leads to a triple increase in asymptomatic herpes, meaning that patients are acquiring the disease, yet are not displaying outbreaks that are detectable. Prevalence of herpes increases with age and number of sexual partners and is greatest amongst women than men—21% of women versus 12% of men. Various clinical categories of herpes infections are included in a table below for healthcare providers to communicate with each other in similar terms regarding the patient's herpes presentation. This table is under the assumption that the patient has had blood testing for HSV (rarely done in current practice) and, therefore, when a positive culture is obtained from a patient's sore, there are HSV antibodies from blood testing to compare to.

If I have lost you at this point, do not worry! I offer underneath this table a real-life interpretation of what is captured.

Clinical designation of genital herpes simplex virus infection (HSV)

Primary genital HSV infection
Antibodies to both HSV-1 and HSV-2 are absent at the time the patient acquires genital HSV due to HSV-1 or HSV-2
Nonprimary first episode genital HSV infection
Acquisition of genital HSV-2 with preexisting antibodies to HSV-1
or
Acquisition of genital HSV-1 with preexisting antibodies to HSV-2*
Recurrent genital HSV infection
Reactivation of genital HSV in which the HSV type recovered from the lesion is the same type as antibodies in the serum

* This occurs extremely rarely.

UpToDate

Simplified Clinical Scenario Explanation of the table above:
- Primary Genital HSV infection:
  - Patient does not have a history of HSV. Testing is done after an exposure and blood test or culture converts to having either HSV 1 or HSV 2 positive results.
    - I.e. Patrick + me in college: my first genital lesion cultured positive for HSV 1 via oral sex
- Nonprimary first episode genital HSV infection:
  - Patient has positive HSV 1 blood test results and receives a positive HSV 2 genital culture OR (extremely rare) patient has positive HSV 2 blood test results and received positive HSV 1 genital culture. It is nonprimary because HSV is already detected in the blood.
    - I.e. Seth + me: I had already tested positive for HSV 1 from college but then was positive for HSV 2 from Seth
- Recurrent genital HSV infection:
  - Patient has known positive HSV blood test results and has a recurrent outbreak of the same HSV strain from a positive genital culture. (This would be me now after my initial outbreak)

In the United States, genital herpes related to HSV 1 or HSV 2 infection is reported to be the most common ulcerative sexually transmitted infections followed by syphilis; chancroid is a distant third, often in the context of small focused outbreaks[13]. The prevalence varies country to country.

---

[13] Centers for Disease Control and Prevention, Division of Sexually Transmitted Diseases. Sexually Transmitted Diseases Surveillance, Other Sexually Transmitted Diseases, 2007. www.cdc.gov/std/stats07/tables.htm (Accessed on September 30, 2009).

*I understand HSV 2 is transmitted sexually, but how can
I acquire HSV 1 if it generally oral lesions?*[14]

HSV 1 is transmitted from person-to-person via herpetic lesions
or oral secretions containing HSV 1 during close contact (simply,
kissing someone or being kissed by someone who has oral
herpes). In various studies, HSV was cultured from 81–88% of
vesicles, 34% of ulcers or crusts, and from the saliva in 3.6–25%
of patients with a positive history or serology. 2–9% of adults
and 5-8% of children were asymptomatic salivary excretors of
HSV 1.[15] The viral titer[16] is 100 to 100 times greater when lesions
are present; as a result, transmission is much more likely when
the patient is symptomatic.[17]

*Can I be a herpes carrier and give it to people I have been
sexually active with? Or, can I be a herpes carrier and not
know for many years?*

Absolutely. Herpes can be asymptomatic and subclinical.
There can be viral shedding even though there is no evidence
of a lesion. One study estimates 0.65-15% of adults may be
excreting HSV 1 or HSV 2 at any time. Only after that first

[14] Douglas RG Jr, Couch RB. A prospective study of chronic herpes simplex virus
infection and recurrent herpes labialis in humans. J Immunol. 1970; 104(2):289.
Spruance SL, Overall JC Jr, Kern ER, Krueger GG, Pliam V, Miller W. The natural history of recurrent herpes simplex labialis: implications for antiviral therapy. N Engl J
Med. 1977; 297(2):69.
Young SK, Rowe NH, Buchanan RA. A clinical study for the control of facial muco-
cutaneous herpes virus infections. I. Characterization of natural history in a professional school population. Oral Surg Oral Med Oral Pathol. 1976; 41(4):498.
[15] Corey L, Spear PG. Infections with herpes simplex viruses (1). N Engl J Med.
1986; 314(11):686.
[16] Viral titer: A titer is a way of expressing concentration. A viral titer is the lowest
concentration of virus that still infects cells. In this instance, the virus amount is
greater when lesions are present.
[17] Corey L, Spear PG. Infections with herpes simplex viruses (1). N Engl J Med. 1986;
314(11):686.

lesion occurs do most people seek evaluation and find out the positive result. It is very common in my practice to have patients who have had the infection for many years and not have a first outbreak until many years later. It is important not to blame your current partner for withholding STI history because it is possible that you may have acquired the infection from someone in your past, not necessarily this current partner.

How do I know I have herpes? What does the lesion look like?

Most people with herpes either have no or very mild symptoms and a person may not even notice the mild symptoms. Genital herpes sores classically appear as one or a cluster of shallow, tender blisters on or around the genitalia, rectum or mouth. The blisters break and leave painful sores that may take a week to heal. These ulcers may coalesce into one large ulcer. Sometimes the ulcers present as "kissing lesions," first showing on one side of the labia and then infecting the other labia where the skin touches. It is not uncommon when people come in for a first outbreak to say, "I got one and then I noticed on the other side there was another one in the exact same spot." These ulcers can get secondary infections so evaluation is important. It is important that when you do touch the sore to immediately wash your hands thoroughly so you can avoid spreading the infection.[18]

Herpes can be associated with flu-like symptoms—patients can have fever, headaches, local pain and itching, body aches, swollen or tender groin[19] lymph nodes.

[18] American College of Obstetricians and Gynecologists. Gynecological Herpes Simplex Virus Infections. ACOG Practice Bulletin No. 57.
[19] Groin—the fold or hollow on either side of the front of the body where the thigh joins the abdomen.

Ulcerations can also present for other diseases. This list can be split into infectious or noninfectious processes.

Infectious
- Syphilis: this ulceration is painless, indurated, and has a clean base to the ulcer or chancre. This is separated from herpes with a blood test for syphilis.
- Chancroid: deeply formed ulceration causing a painful groin infection of the lymph nodes. This is caused by highly infectious bacteria called *Haemophilus ducreyi*.

Noninfectious
- Yeast infection[20]: irritation from a yeast infection causes scratching and a healing scratch can present like an ulceration. Evaluation in the office to see if a yeast infection is present, as well as viral culture is appropriate in this case.
- Inflammatory bowel disease: is a group of inflammatory conditions of the colon and small intestine. Crohn's disease and ulcerative colitis are principal types of inflammatory bowel disease. Crohn's disease can also affect the mouth, esophagus, stomach, and anus, whereas ulcerative colitis primarily affects the colon and rectum.
- Aphthous ulcers: aka canker sores that are painful, rounded, small ulcerations and limit eating. Typically spontaneously heal within 1-3 weeks.
- Behcet's ulcers: recurrent painful oral and genital ulcers (most specific manifestation) along with multiple other systemic manifestations due to a vascular inflammatory disease.
- Skin cancer, local trauma, ingrown hairs (aka folliculitis) from waxing or shaving, pimples, and hemorrhoids can also present as skin irritations.

---

[20] AKA candidiasis

Viral culture is the standard diagnostic method for isolating HSV from genital lesions to give the diagnosis of genital herpes. The diagnosis yield is the highest in the earliest stage of the disease when the lesion is fluid-filled and a culture can be obtained. Thus, the encouragement is for patients to be evaluated within the first few days; however, it can be sensitive and painful to culture. Overall sensitivity of viral genital lesions is only ~50%. When the lesion begins to heal, the viral load decreases, and it can be difficult to obtain an accurate result. In this instance, the vesicle can be unroofed (remove the top layer of the scar) and the ulcer underneath sampled. Because this was obtained when the lesion started to heal, a negative result does not necessarily clear someone from the diagnosis.

Blood testing

Clinical scenario: Patient to provider: "My boyfriend tested positive by blood test for herpes. He nor I have ever had a genital outbreak. Will you test me to see if he gave it to me?"

Serologic blood testing is an antiquated method of testing that was historically done in the past. The thought process behind blood testing is that it results in detection of type specific antibodies that develop in the first weeks after an infection and persist indefinitely. However, in one study of 164 adults with confirmed primary genital HSV infection, only 40 (24%) had HSV DNA detected in blood work.

The basic rule of medicine is to order a laboratory test or radiology evaluation if the clinician believes the result will change the management or the outcome. Ultimately, the patient wants the answer to the question: "Do I have genital herpes or do I not?" If this patient tests positive for either HSV 1 or HSV 2 via blood, it will not give us further information. We will wait for a positive genital outbreak to know for certain.

Serologic blood testing for HSV 1 and HSV 2 can be used to:
- Diagnose a patient with a history of genital lesions who did not have a diagnostic workup
- Diagnose a past or present HSV infection in a patient with an atypical presentation
- Determine susceptibility of a sexual partner of a patient with documented culture positive genital HSV infection

The relatively high seroprevalence[21] rate of HSV 2 in the US (22% in persons ≥12yrs of age between 1988 and 1994) and the risk of transmission to sexual partners has raised the question of whether serology screening may be justified in asymptomatic (showing no evidence of disease) sexually active individuals. At present, routine blood testing for HSV 2 is NOT recommended because there may be a relatively high false positive rate in low-risk populations. False positive equates to "False Alarm". If a patient has a genital lesion that is HSV positive, the patient has the clinical diagnosis of herpes based on the positive culture, not on blood testing alone.

If I commonly get cold sores on my lips, does that mean I have herpes?

Cold sores and canker sores are terms often confused with each other, but they are not the same.
- Cold sores, AKA fever blisters, are caused by HSV 1. These sores typically appear outside the mouth, usually under the nose, around the lips, or under the chin.

---

[21] Seroprevalence: number of people in a population who test positive for a specific disease based on serology (blood serum) specimens.

- Canker sores, AKA aphthous ulcers, are caused by stress or tissue injury. Certain foods (acidic fruits and vegetables), braces, sharp foods, or tooth surfaces can trigger canker sores. Impaired immune system and nutritional problems may also manifest canker sores.

Do resistant antibodies exist?[22]

There is a relatively rare HSV 2 resistance to Acyclovir in patients who are on chronic antiviral medication suppression. The rate was 0.18% to 0.32%. Even if there is drug resistance to herpes, it can be cleared normally without clinical outcomes.

There has been some drug resistance observed in HIV positive patients in long-term therapy.[23]

Do I have an increased risk of HIV?

The literature demonstrates with HSV 2 there can be an increased risk of contracting HIV. Tiny breaks in the genital and anal area due to herpes can provide entry into the body. The herpes infection is attracted to the type of cells that HIV infects in the genital area, so this can increase the chance of HIV if exposed to it.

---

[22] Danve-Szatanek C, Aymard M, Thouvenot D, Morfin F, Agius G, Bertin I, Billaudel S, Chanzy B, Coste-Burel M, Finkielsztejn L, Fleury H, Hadou T, Henquell C, Lafeuille H, Lafon ME, Le Faou A, Legrand MC, Maille L, Mengelle C, Morand P, Morinet F, Nicand E, Omar S, Picard B, Pozzetto B, Puel J, Raoult D, Scieux C, Segondy M, Seigneurin JM, Teyssou R, Zandotti C. Surveillance network for herpes simplex virus resistance to antiviral drugs: 3-year follow-up. J Clin Microbiol. 2004; 42(1):242.
[23] Reyes M, Shaik NS, Graber JM, Nisenbaum R, Wetherall NT, Fukuda K, Reeves WC, Task Force on Herpes Simplex Virus Resistance. Acyclovir-resistant genital herpes among persons attending sexually transmitted disease and human immunodeficiency virus clinics. Arch Intern Med. 2003; 163(1):76.

Is herpes related to shingles?

I acquired shingles a few months ago during a stressful time in my life, and one of my physician colleagues jokingly asked me, "How's your herpes doing?" At first, I was stunned because I thought he had found out my STI history before I admitted it to him, but then I realized he was joking and was referring to the microbiology tree learned in medical school.

Herpesviridae is a large family of DNA viruses that cause latent diseases in humans. The members of this family are known as herpesviruses. The family name is derived from the Greek word *herpein* ("to creep"), referring to the latent, recurring infections typical of this group of viruses. At least five species of herpesviridae are extremely widespread among humans.

- HSV 1 and HSV 2—both cause orolabial herpes and genital herpes
- Varicella zoster virus—causes chickenpox and shingles
- Epstein Barr virus—causes mononucleosis ("mono")
- Cytomegalovirus

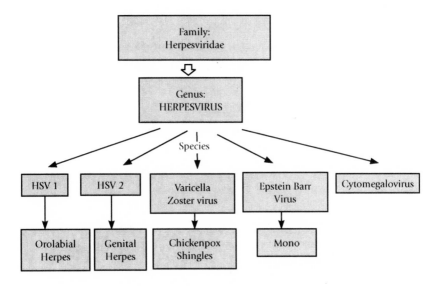

More than 90% of adults have been infected with at least one of these, and a latent form of the virus remains in most people.[24] In total, there are 8 herpesvirus types that infect humans: herpes simplex viruses 1 and 2, varicella-zoster virus, EBV (Epstein-Barr virus), human cytomegalovirus, human herpesvirus 6, human herpesvirus 7, and Kaposi's sarcoma-associated herpesvirus.

Chickenpox exposure is highly contagious and generally occurs in childhood. This infection is characterized by vesicular lesions on the face, trunk, and extremities in various stages. The varicella zoster virus acts in the same way as herpes in that it can lay dormant in the spinal cord. The latent virus infection in the spinal cord, in the sensory ganglion and the nervous system can be reactivated causing Shingles. This is an ailment causing painful, one-sided vesicles or blisters that erupt on a certain skin dermatome on one side of the body or the other.

What is the average incubation period for herpes?

The incubation period is the time elapsed between exposure and when symptoms and signs are first apparent. In this period, the organism is replicating to a threshold necessary to produce symptoms in the patient. The average incubation period after herpes exposure is 4 days (range, 2 to 12).

Transmission of herpes occurs quickly in new relationships. In one study, among 199 of newly acquired genital herpes, the median duration of a sexual relationship to exposure was 3.5 months, and that ranged 1.5 to 10 months, or a median number

---

[24] Staras SA, Dollard SC, Radford KW, Flanders WD, Pass RF, Cannon MJ (November 2006). "Seroprevalence of cytomegalovirus infection in the United States, 1988–1994". Clin. Infect. Dis. 43(9):1143–51.

Chayavichitsilp P, Buckwalter JV, Krakowski AC, Friedlander SF (April 2009). "Herpes simplex". Pediatr Rev 30(4):119–29; quiz 130.

of sex acts before transmission was 40.[25] Condom use was also noted to be infrequent—50% during first intercourse, 20% during last intercourse before diagnosis. The median time of infection was greater in participants whose partners informed them they had herpes than those partners who did not—270 days versus 60 days. Another study evaluating 144 sexual couples found the rate of acquiring genital herpes was higher in females negative for HSV 1 and HSV 2 (32%) than those with preexisting HSV 1 (9%).

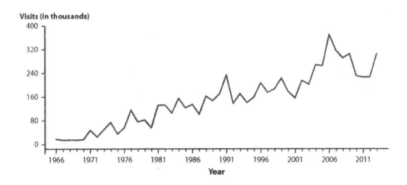

This graph[26] shows the dramatic spike in diagnosis of herpes from 1999 until 2003.

How does online dating play a role in the spread of STDs?

According to *The Washington Post*[27] in 2015, research on whether or not dating apps have killed courtship and irrevocably altered romance as we know it is largely inconclusive. The correlation between online and mobile dating and increased rates of STI

[25] Wald A, Krantz E, Selke S, et al. Knowledge of partners' genital herpes protects against herpes simplex virus type 2 acquisition. J Infect Dis 2006; 194:42.

[26] http://www.cdc.gov/std/stats14/figures/53.htm

[27] https://www.washingtonpost.com/news/morning-mix/wp/2015/09/29/billboards-linking-tinder-to-stds-are-latest-battleground-in-online-dating-wars. Retrieved May 23, 2016.

transmissions was more compelling, at least on a state-by-state basis. In Utah, there were huge increases since 2011 in the number of gonorrhea diagnoses—700% for women, nearly 300% for men. The links between STI rates and app use in Utah are still anecdotal however apps make casual, anonymous encounters easier, and it can be impossible to find one-night stand partners again. The most conclusive evidence linking the Internet to STI rates is a much cited 2013 study that found that the introduction of Craigslist to 33 states across the country led to a 15% increase in HIV rates. It has been difficult to find data specific for herpes mostly because herpes is not reportable to the state once positive. However we can conclude generally given the large amount if undiagnosed asymptomatic herpes in the community that online dating can spread the virus exponentially.

Dating is often fraught with uncertainty and self-consciousness. Tailored websites for those with STIs, such as herpes and HPV[28] have been created. These specialized dating websites offer a safe space for those who wish to avoid the stigmas of mainstream society. Often this removes the terror of telling a new partner about their STI. Even if you are let down politely, it still affects your self-confidence. Some dating site skeptics of this niche believe these sites are based on the fundamental principle of being different and need to find another individual that is different to date. Some believe that these sites can also give a false impression that just because you have the same STI, unprotected sex is safe.[29]

---

[28] HPV: Human Papilloma Virus is the most common sexually transmitted infection (STI). HPV is a different virus than HIV and HSV. HPV is so common that nearly all sexually active men and women get it at some point in their lives. There are many different types of HPV. Some types can cause health problems including genital warts and cancers.
[29] "Online dating for people with sexually transmitted infections" BBC News Magazine, 28 March 2013. Retrieved 5/23/16.
http://www.bbc.com/news/magazine-21955126

Is it possible to be misdiagnosed with herpes?

Clinical scenario:

Patient: "It's very interesting. Every single time I garden, every year, I seem to get these outbreaks vaginally. I'm no longer with my husband; he passed away 10 years ago, but it always just seems to happen. And it goes away on its own. I realize I am coming in 3 days after it recurred, but is this something I should have come in sooner for?" My examination of this 70-year-old patient showed ulcerations on both sides of her labia, which is where these lesions present and regress spontaneously. Given that these lesions are recurrent, I completed a herpes culture by unroofing the scab on the lesion and sent the culture to the lab. A culture can take ~48 hours to return, depending on the lab, so I offered to treat her with antiviral medications. I suspected that the culture may come back negative because it has been too long, but it was better to go ahead and start treatment than to wait. I also obtained a syphilis blood test, which came back negative and informed her if the lesions did not get better with the antivirals, to come back to the office for a biopsy to rule out vulvar skin cancer.

The herpes culture and syphilis test came back negative. When I notified the patient, she informed me that when she started to take the antivirals, her ulcerations got better. Since she was improving with the antivirals, it was better to continue the medication course than stop. I offered a vulvar biopsy which she declined. I informed her to return when she first sees the sign of the outbreak so we can obtain a culture.

In this patient interaction, one could say that she was misdiagnosed because her culture came back negative. However, due to the fact that she improved on antiviral medication and her culture was obtained several days after the onset of the outbreak, this is more of an unknown/'to be determined' case until the next outbreak.

HERPES AND PREGNANCY

Can I get safely pregnant if I have herpes?

Herpes is treatable in pregnancy; however, this skin condition can have serious health consequences for a woman who becomes pregnant and whose partner failed to disclose the herpes infection. Patients come to me and ask, "Is it okay if I get pregnant?" "Is it bad for my baby?" My response is an emphatic: "Go for it! Have a baby! There are medications you can take to prevent passing the virus to your child. If joy will come from having a child, we can treat your herpes preventatively. There is no reason for that to stop life at all!"

Clinical scenario: One of my patients learned she contracted HSV 2 from her former husband, her first and only partner, shortly after giving birth to their first child. The daughter started having seizures within the first week of life and through testing was determined to have herpetic encephalitis, a condition that affects the human nervous system caused by HSV. Her husband had been dishonest about his medical history, and while her daughter received IV treatment, she has had many medical issues such as blindness, abnormal bone growth, and is nonverbal. In subsequent pregnancies, my patient took antiviral medication starting at 36 weeks and has since delivered healthy children with no long-term deficits.

If I get pregnant, will my child get it?

Suppressive antiviral treatment is recommended at 36 weeks until after delivery, which reduces the risk of lesions at delivery. The treatment decreases the risk of severe and prolonged symptoms and complicated new infections for the mother. The medication is safe for the baby and the mother. Acyclovir, which is used to treat herpes, is safe during pregnancy in both animal and human data, even in the first trimester and in all stages of the pregnancy. Several other medications exist. Valacyclovir is reassuring in pregnancy, although the data is limited. Famciclovir is another antiviral medication that does not have any human data at this time.

If someone is pregnant and has a primary infection, the treatment is Acyclovir, 400 mg three times a day for seven to 10 days. The treatment may be extended if the healing is incomplete. Intravenous (IV) Acyclovir is indicated in severe infections, and although suppression therapy markedly reduces the frequency of symptom disease in asymptomatic viral shedding, the effect on incidence of neonatal[30] herpes is not known.

There are no studies examining the utility of suppression treatment with blood positive type 2 who do not have confirmation of genital outbreak. In these situations, antiviral therapy is not recommended.

Clinical scenario: "My boyfriend is positive for genital herpes. I have never had a genital outbreak. Should I be on suppression at 36 weeks?" In this scenario, the answer would be "no," because there is no diagnosed confirmed positive culture of a genital sore.[31]

Clinical scenario: "I have a history of recurrent herpes. I am scared that my baby is going to get it. Go ahead and do a prophylactic C-section on me. Please do a C-section even though I don't have symptoms." If there is no evidence or symptoms of an active lesion, the risk of neonatal herpes is very low. It is important to consider the risks versus benefit in all aspects of your health. The risk of surgery is greater than the benefit of a possible herpes infection being transmitted to the fetus.

---

[30] Neonatal: of or relating to newborn children.
[31] Workowski KA, Bolan GA. Sexually transmitted diseases treatment guidelines, 2015. Centers for Disease Control and Prevention, MMWR Recomm Rep. 2015; 64(RR-03):1.

Am I managed differently in labor because I have herpes?

During labor, the obstetricians prefer to avoid breaks in the fetal skin because that can be a potential risk factor for neonatal herpes. Breaks in the fetal skin can occur from instruments like a vacuum/forceps to expedite a vaginal delivery, or incidental laceration from a scalpel. However, in the end, the clinical situation will be judged by the person taking care of you and the risks and benefits weighed.

Clinical scenario: The mother-to-be is 39 weeks at time of delivery, has a history of herpes, but has been on Acyclovir since 36 weeks, and is asymptomatic of any lesions. She has been pushing for 2 hours and the baby is crowning. The baby's heart rate decelerates for several minutes, and an expedited delivery is recommended. The obstetrician recommends a vacuum delivery, given fetal intolerance to labor, and the mother agrees. Baby is delivered successfully without complications.

Certain high-risk situations, such as a patient with a history of herpes who is in preterm labor or has preterm premature rupture of membranes, are out of the scope of this book; however, there are treatments with Acyclovir to prevent neonatal transmission.

Can a mother pass herpes through the vaginal birthing process of a baby?[32]

Yes. If a woman has a previous diagnosis of herpes and is pregnant, the major concern is maternal HSV herpes infection transmitted to the fetus. The transmission can occur during delivery. Disease within the uterus is rare and the risk of transmission in the placenta is low. However, if the mother has an open lesion on the vulva, vagina, cervix, rectum and/or

---

[32] ACOG Practice Bulletin. Clinical management guidelines for obstetrician-gynecologists. No. 82 June 2007. Management of herpes in pregnancy. ACOG Committee on Practice Bulletins Obstet Gynecol. 2007 Jun; 109(6):1489–98.

perineal area, there is viral shedding that can occur. Even if the mother does not have a lesion or is asymptomatic, viral shedding can occur. Therefore, when the baby is in contact with the virus during labor and delivery, there is an increased risk of exposure.[33]

The concentration and duration of viral shedding is higher when someone has a first infection versus a recurrent infection. The risk of spreading the infection to the baby is highest in women who are having their first outbreak in or near their time of delivery. This is why taking antiviral medication during pregnancy is important to decrease the risk of shedding during labor.

Patients who present to labor and delivery with symptoms such as tingling, numbness, or a herpes outbreak at the time of labor are automatically delivered via Cesarean section to decrease exposure of the baby with a vaginal route.

Clinical scenario: Patient past her due date with a history of herpes presents to Labor and Delivery stating, "I have some tingling and pain, but I don't think I have an outbreak. I did not start my Acyclovir like my OB recommended." In this instance, proceeding with a C-section is recommended because the risk to the baby is still great.[34]

What if I was born with it?

A neonatal infection with herpes occurs in one out of 3,200 to 10,000 live births. Neonatal herpes accounts for 0.2% of fetal hospitalizations and 0.6% in hospital neonatal deaths.

---

[33] Vontver LA, Hickok DE, Brown Z, Reid L, Corey L. Recurrent genital herpes simplex virus infection in pregnancy: infant outcome and frequency of asymptomatic recurrences. Am J Obstet Gynecol. 1982; 143(1):75.

[34] Brown ZA, Wald A, Morrow RA, Selke S, Zeh J, Corey L. Effect of serologic status and cesarean delivery on transmission rates of herpes simplex virus from mother to infant. JAMA. 2003; 289(2):203.

Herpes can be transmitted in utero, which is rare, occurring in one out of 250,000 deliveries. 85% of neonatal infections occur when a baby is exposed to an undiagnosed infection in the vagina. Infections after the baby is born make up 10%. That can happen when a caretaker with an active herpes infection has close contact with a newborn infant. For example, herpes can be passed if someone has an oral outbreak and then was kissing the baby on the eyes.

When a baby gets neonatal herpes, 45% is found in the skin, eyes, and mouth. It is benign at onset, but there can be a high risk of progression to neurologic or disseminated disease if not treated. Baby may have eye watering, may seem to be crying from eye pain, eye redness, ulcerations on the tongue, mouth, and palate. There could be clustering of the vesicle with a red erythematous base around it.

Neonatal herpes involves the central nervous system. It can start from the fetal nose, then go up into the olfactory nerves, and then spread to the brain. That can occur in the second or third week of life, but can occur up to the first six weeks. Usually these babies end up with seizures, lethargy, irritability, tremors, poor feeding, and temperature instability. On physical exam, a full anterior–fontanelle[35] is noted. With neonatal herpes, disseminated disease[36] can occur which is the fourth stage, and then sepsis[37] can occur. It involves multiple organs, requiring admission to the hospital and IV antiviral medication.[38]

---

[35] The anterior fontanelle (bregmatic fontanelle, frontal fontanelle) is the largest fontanelle and is used clinically. The fontanelle allows the skull to deform during birth to ease its passage through the birth canal and for expansion of the brain after birth.

[36] Disseminated disease: A disseminated infection extending beyond its origin and spreading to infect other areas of the body.

[37] Sepsis: A disseminated infection extending beyond its origin and spreading to infect other areas of the body.

[38] Demmler-Harrison GJ. Neonatal herpes simplex virus infection: Clinical features and diagnosis. In: UpToDate, Kaplan SL and Weisman LE (Ed), UpToDate. (Accessed on March 1, 2016.)

Does a primary infection present differently than a recurrent infection?

The clinical presentation can be varied based on the type of infection. Outpatient medical management is preferred; however, treatment is based on the clinical situation. A primary infection is highly variable—it can be one ulceration, multiple painful genital ulcers, or so severe it requires admission to the hospital.

Clinical scenario: 17 year old was evaluated in the emergency room with inability to urinate and was found to have urinary retention secondary to her first primary episode of large herpetic lesions. She had a secondary bacterial infection of the sores and was unable to walk due to swelling and pain. She was started on IV antiviral Acyclovir, as well as IV skin antibiotics. A Foley catheter was placed in her bladder and there was judicious use of lidocaine jelly and ice packs to soothe the sores. She was in the hospital for 4 days.

Recurrent infections are typically less severe and symptoms more mild. A visit to the office is not necessary; because the patient generally understands their presentations, a call to your provider to obtain antiviral medications is reasonable.

Will I live with this forever?

The herpes virus lives indefinitely within the spinal cord and can remain dormant or become reactivated.

Will it get worse as I get older?

Patients with primary herpes should be aware that future outbreaks are expected.

Outbreaks decrease throughout life, both in severity and frequency. Generally, it does not get worse. It is important to recognize when you have the infection so treatment can be started and decrease the duration when symptoms are present.

Chapter Six

TREATMENT OPTIONS

"Hope is being able to see that there is light despite all of the darkness."

— Desmond Tutu

Treatment options: How do I treat herpes outbreaks?

In terms of conventional treatment options, the antiviral medication Acyclovir can prevent or shorten the duration of the signs and symptoms during the period when the patient is taking the medication. There is no cure for herpes, but there is medication available to reduce symptoms and make it less likely that you will spread herpes to another partner.

Initiation of oral antibiotics within 72 hours of lesion appearance may decrease duration and severity of illness by days to weeks. Acyclovir, Famciclovir, and Valacyclovir are efficacious, and dosing and duration is dependent on which agent is chosen. CDC guidelines have standard recommendations on dosaging of these antivirals; please defer to your healthcare provider regarding Acyclovir, Famciclovir, and Valacyclovir dosages. Occasionally, an infection is so severe that IV antiviral medication is required.

Episodic treatment is self-administered antiviral treatment for outbreaks as they arise. When prodromal[39] symptoms, such as tingling, numbness, itching, pain or ulceration, occur prior to the onset of lesions, episodic treatment can be started.

---

[39] An early symptom that might indicate the start of a disease.

If initiated within the first 24 hours, Acyclovir is associated with faster resolution. When my patient's present for their first outbreak, they are informed that if they have future outbreaks they do not need another appointment. Now that they are aware of the symptoms, they can contact via email or phone and request antiviral medication.

The safety of long-term therapy has been demonstrated over six years of continuous treatment. The natural recurrence diminishes over time, whether or not antiviral treatment is given. Like the 70-year-old gardener in my previous story, if she was on antiviral medications, it may or may not decrease the days of an outbreak since she had not treated it for so long.

It is best to speak to your local pharmacist or your medical provider regarding interaction with other medications. In greater than 10% of patients, the largest side effect with Acyclovir is fatigue with the oral pills.

What is daily suppression medication?

Daily antiviral suppression therapy can reduce the likelihood of transmission to partners. With daily suppression medication, there is decreased viral shedding of 50%. Chronic suppression is for those with greater than six outbreaks a year or want to decrease risk of transmission to their partner.

Suppression medication is a topic of discussion on an annual basis. Some patients may choose to discontinue using suppression; however, some people do not want to discontinue due to concern of getting another outbreak. But antiviral treatment is very well tolerated in primary episodic therapy. It is rare to have resistance to the medication, and although studies of chronic suppression have not shown significant toxicity, many studies have limited long-term follow-up of less than one year.

In the absence of suppressive antiviral therapy, the median occurrence rate after a first episode of herpes is four per year, with 40% having less than six recurrences in a year. Twenty percent (20%) had more than 10 within the first year. Over time, the recurrence generally decreases in number. With recurrent infections, lesions may be asymptomatic, few in number, and atypical in appearance. Fissures or vulva irritation, itching, or pain may be how they present, particularly in women.

The treatment strategy for recurrent disease is influenced by the frequency of episodes, severity of signs and symptoms, and the risk of viral transmission to uninfected sexual partners.

How do I choose between episodic (as needed) and chronic (everyday) suppression?

A study done on quality of life found being on chronic suppressive therapy was superior. The probability of recurrence was 78% lower with suppression. Treatment satisfaction existed and there was no serious toxicity.[40]

The choice of episodic versus chronic suppressive therapy should be individualized to the patient's preference. I usually ask patients, "Would you like to call in and just get medication when you have an episode, or would you prefer to take something every day?" Some patients do not want to take daily medication; perhaps they are not in a long-term relationship, find the medication costly and not covered by insurance, or daily pills a nuisance.

Convenience, the frequency of occurrence, and adherence to daily dosing can be burdensome. Some patients for psychosocial considerations will rely on chronic suppression because it gives them less stress and anxiety. Some do not want to know that they have the virus due to minimal outbreaks; others take the medicine like a daily multivitamin and do not think twice.

[40] Fife KH, Almekinder J, Ofner S. A comparison of one year of episodic or suppressive treatment of recurrent genital herpes with valacyclovir. Sex Transm Dis. 2007; 34(5):297.

Is there a natural way of treating herpes if you do not want to use traditional medicine?

Some patients use lysine supplements to curb any herpes outbreaks. Increasing lysine in the diet is a method to speed recovery and reduce the chance of recurrent outbreaks. Lysine rich foods are fish, chicken, eggs, and potatoes. It is recommended to take high doses of lysine in a short amount of time.

Repetitively in the office, I recommend a healthy diet and exercise to all my patients—fruits, vegetables, antioxidants, and multivitamins. My basis of this endorsement is the more we can boost our immune systems by treating ourselves well, decreasing stress, taking time for ourselves, and making ourselves a priority—those practices will decrease infection. I admit I do not exercise this ALL of the time. But, forgive a weak moment and spend the majority of time eating well. Having one cheat day a week helps quiet cravings, and being realistic can be the key to success. Spend 90% of the time following the diet and use the 10% for cautious splurge meals. It is an investment in yourself for life longevity and decrease in herpes outbreaks.

Other treatments exist to decrease the severity of the first episode and the local pain that is associated with it. A topical anesthetic like lidocaine jelly works well and can be bought over the counter or exists in prescription strength from your clinician. Soaking in sitz baths has been found to soothe the sores as well as keep the area clean to prevent secondary infections. A sitz bath is created with warm water with Epsom salts dissolved in the water. I recommend soaking for approximately 15 minutes two to three times a day. Baby aspirin, Tylenol, or Ibuprofen can help ease the pain from the symptoms. Wearing loose cotton underwear during the day and going without at night can help with healing.

Scientists have studied herbal extracts and nutritional supplements. Some studies are promising; others are discouraging. There is not one treatment other than antivirals that has shown great promise.

What about the effects of exercise on herpes?

Exercise has been applauded as a great way to maintain health and longevity. I will not belabor the point as we have the recommendation to exercise thrown at us daily. However exercise is a great way to clear toxins. The increased breathing that occurs during exercise is a wonderful way to oxygenate the organs of the body and remove toxins. The skin is our greatest elimination organ. Perspiration and sweating through increased heart rate is a valuable tool. Increased hydration (with water!) helps with elimination of further toxins.

What are the effects of nutrition on herpes and mental health?

Food affects both our physical and mental health. Research linking diet and mental health shows that food, along with other factors, plays an important contributing role in the development, managements and prevention of specific mental health problems, such as depression, schizophrenia, ADHD, and Alzheimer's disease.

The saying "you are what you eat" has truth in it. Most of us have likely experienced when certain foods make us feel fatigued or sluggish after eating. I affectionately call this phenomena my "food coma," a great way to induce an afternoon nap. Thanksgiving meals have a remarkable way of creating discomfort and fatigue, contrasted with a morning fruit and protein smoothie that makes me feel energized and light.

In 2004, Morgan Spurlock's extreme documentary called "Super Size Me" extremely depicted the obesity epidemic, as

well as how food can make someone feel. He ate solely at
McDonald's three times a day for 30 days. If he was offered to
"super size" a meal, his obligated answer was "Yes." He restricted
himself to no physical activity limiting himself to 5,000 steps a
day (approximately 2.5 miles).

Not only did he gain weight, increase his cholesterol and
blood pressure, he found he suffered from massive headaches,
lethargy and had never been so depressed in his life. And this
was only by mid month!

Simply put, food is fuel and the kinds of foods and drinks
consumed determine the types of nutrients in your system.
These nutrients impact how well your mind and body are able
to function. Expending energy to clear your body of toxins
rather than using it to digest unhealthy food seems like a better
use of energy.

Is there a cure for herpes?

There is no vaccine available that protects against type 1 or
type 2. Researchers have focused on the development of a
preventative and/or therapeutic vaccine for herpes, but studies
have not been successful.[41] Several therapeutic vaccine trials

[41] Belshe RB, Leone PA, Bernstein DI, Wald A, Levin MJ, Stapleton JT, Gorfinkel I, Morrow RL, Ewell MG, Stokes-Riner A, Dubin G, Heineman TC, Schulte JM, Deal CD, Herpevac Trial for Women. Efficacy results of a trial of a herpes simplex vaccine. N Engl J Med. 2012 Jan; 366(1):34–43.

Straus SE, Wald A, Kost RG, McKenzie R, Langenberg AG, Hohman P, Lekstrom J, Cox E, Nakamura M, Sekulovich R, Izu A, Dekker C, Corey L. Immunotherapy of recurrent genital herpes with recombinant herpes simplex virus type 2 glycoproteins D and B: results of a placebo-controlled vaccine trial. J Infect Dis. 1997; 176(5):1129.

Straus SE, Corey L, Burke RL, Savarese B, Barnum G, Krause PR, Kost RG, Meier JL, Sekulovich R, Adair SF. Placebo-controlled trial of vaccination with recombinant glycoprotein D of herpes simplex virus type 2 for immunotherapy of genital herpes. Lancet. 1994; 343(8911):1460.

de Bruyn G, Vargas-Cortez M, Warren T, Tyring SK, Fife KH, Lalezari J, Brady RC, Shahmanesh M, Kinghorn G, Beutner KR, Patel R, Drehobl MA, Horner P, Kurtz TO, McDermott S, Wald A, Corey L. A randomized controlled trial of a replication defective (gH deletion) herpes simplex virus vaccine for the treatment of recurrent genital herpes among immunocompetent subjects. Vaccine. 2006; 24(7):914.

have also been conducted to 'boost' natural immunity in prior HSV 2 infections to decrease reoccurrences but further studies are ongoing to optimize dose, dose regime and impact on recurrence.[42]

Is there a preventative contraceptive?

No. Consistent condom use is a safe sex recommendation. Condoms do not protect from all STIs, but it will hopefully protect the majority of exposures.

[42] Rouse BT, Kaistha SD. A tale of 2 alpha-herpesviruses: lessons for vaccinologists. Clin Infect Dis. 2006; 42(6):810.

Chapter Seven

EMOTIONAL TURMOIL: WHAT DID I DO TO DESERVE THIS?

UNFORTUNATELY, WE CANNOT know how or when herpes was acquired unless there was only one physical contact with one other person. If a person has more than one partner, herpes could have been acquired from your first kiss, first oral sex, first genital intercourse, etc. As providers in the office, we have no clue who the infection came from; our intent is to diagnose the ulcerations and treat.

Do I need to tell every person that I have ever been with in the past?

This would be a very personal decision because some people need that closure and feel responsible for doing due diligence. Moving forward, I encourage informing future partners. It is in the best interest in the health for yourself and the community.

I feel like I will never be loved again because of this; how do I cope?

These are your own valid emotions; please do not dismiss them. Why do you think you cannot be loved? What is the source of that lack of love? Hopefully, through this book, people will realize that there are tools they can use that can show how incredible they are. Once I started doing internal work, all of a sudden it did not matter if I had a partner or not; what mattered is that I love myself as I am. This important perspective shows it may not necessarily be that you need to love somebody else, but I do recommend that you learn to love yourself.

Susannah is a 45-year-old distraught patient who presented to me diagnosed with genital warts, as well as genital herpes. She came to my office a few times for evaluation to ensure she did not concurrently acquire a chlamydia infection or bacterial vaginosis, as well. Evaluation of the suspicious "genital wart" ascertained folliculitis[43] from shaving. Rightfully histrionic, she believed her body and her partner failed her. I reassured her she did not have a simultaneous infection, and I began feeling that she needed someone to talk to. She had been with her partner her whole life but just recently started getting these outbreaks. She admits swearing off of sex completely. In the three months after I saw her, she informed her partner, "NO. I refuse to be active with you in any sort of way."

She felt that he gave it to her since she had two partners in her whole life. I attempted to inform her of the facts of her diagnoses and she felt, "It doesn't matter. I don't want to have sex anymore." I admire her power stance but also believe her to be running away. Perhaps this was her way of coping and controlling the situation. I cautioned her of the desire for belonging, love, and affection as a potent force that shapes various aspects of a person's life. Companionship is fueled by the need to love and be loved. She can certainly consciously choose against companionship at this time, but if Susannah could learn to forgive and love herself, I suspect she could forgive and love her partner again.

"A ship is safe in harbor, but that's not what ships are for."

— William G.T. Shedd

---

[43] Folliculitis: inflammation or infection of the skin follicle.

*"You have been criticizing yourself for years, and it hasn't worked. Try
approving of yourself and see what happens."*

— Louise L. Hay

But I used protection, how did this happen?

While condoms can protect against most STDs and pregnancy,
they do not cover all skin areas that can be exposed. If there is
a visible outbreak, the vesicular fluid can rupture and infect the
skin cells that are present.

What if I never have another outbreak, do I still need to tell people?

Yes, because of those tiny skin outbreaks and the fact that viral
shedding can always occur. In my dating instances, even if I was
not sexually active with these men at that point, I did tell them
because if it was leading in that direction, they needed to know.
If they are not prepared for the possibility of acquiring herpes,
I wanted to be respectful of their desires. Neither of us wastes
each other's time. Why put more effort into something if their
end point is not going to be your end point?

I would recommend telling people that you are intimate with.
It is up to you if you want to tell your immediate and extended
family. Once you have a comfort level and feel steady there,
your openness may guide you to tell others without hesitation.

Is my sex life over?

Clinical scenario: Landon was raised in a devout Latter-Day Saint
(LDS) (Mormon) home; and when he turned 19, he went on a
two year mission for the church. When he came home, he dated
many LDS women, hoping to find someone to marry in the
Mormon temple for "time and all eternity." After a few years of
disappointment, he started dating outside the church and fell

in love with a woman. They had intercourse a few times, but Landon's guilty conscience led him to confess to the church Elders that he had "sinned" and wanted to repent. He was excommunicated from the church. About that time, Landon had his first outbreak of herpetic lesions. He took it as a sign that God was punishing him and he could never be forgiven. Now in his 70s, Landon has never married, probably because shortly after meeting a new woman, he shamefully confides to her, "You probably don't want to get too close to me. I have herpes."

Your sex life is absolutely not over. A healthy sex life is attainable and does not need to be stopped in any way. If you are open and honest, the intimacy can be that much greater. Mating is a natural desire, and there is no reason to deny yourself that happiness due to herpes. You now understand the facts about herpes, the willingness of partners to accept you with herpes, and the common prevalence of herpes; herpes does not have to crumble you.

Should I have sex when I have an outbreak?

No. The viral shedding is at its peak, so waiting until the episode is over would be ideal. If it is a genital outbreak, kissing may be acceptable, but I do not recommend direct contact with the lesion.

Will my partner know if I don't tell?

No. The ulceration is really the only way to tell. Outbreaks do not cause skin scarring so your partner will not know, but it would be in your best interest if you desire to tell them.

You said 'your partner will not know if you don't tell them,' so why should I tell them?

Despite the fact that people read this book, I realize I may not convince readers to be honest and tell their partners.

I understand because I have spent 10+ years exactly where you are. Out of respect for others, it is proper sexual conduct to be honest, particularly when involving someone else's health. Perhaps it is just not time or safe for you, and that is understandable. I encourage seeking support, either through this book, or through friends, religious groups, family, certified therapists, etc. It may not feel like it in the beginning, but if you are dating, perhaps this partner does not want to be with you, but the next partner could be a greater match for you. The universe/God helps those who help themselves.

What if I don't want to have the talk?

You do not have to; no one is forcing you. However, the truth is the truth. There is a power in choice, and I prefer to have a partner actively choose to be with me than being cajoled, manipulated, or duped. The truth is often the most simple, refined answer and is the most direct point between a question and an answer. It is very obvious in retrospect but can take great courage to speak the truth.

These situations do not hurt us; they will not kill you. It is a difficult conversation, but it is one that will get easier and easier every time it is done. You can whisper to yourself internally: "This situation is okay. I am uncomfortable. I don't like the way this makes me feel." Sitting in uncomfortable situations are times when maximum growth can occur.

Pop Culture reference (I was watching the movie while writing this book): At the beginning of the movie *Mr. and Mrs. Smith,* the restrained and proper main characters played by Brad Pitt and Angelina Jolie span to a counseling session where they ask the therapist, "There is a huge space between us, and it just keeps filling with everything we don't say to each other. What's that called?" The counselor replies, "Marriage." Through the course of the movie, Brad and Angelina realize they are skilled assassins pitted to kill each other and their true chemistry flies. This is a grand movie example of when a whole big background exists and once a common ground, honesty, and connection is realized, the relationship grows deeper.

What if I am not really sure I have herpes?

You can express simply that. It is better to be safe than keep your partner in the dark. The conversation may look like, "I went to the doctor; they think they saw something. I'm still waiting for a culture so we will have to wait and see. We should abstain from sexual contact until then." I cannot predict your partner's emotion, but hopefully your partner reflects back respect and concern for your wellbeing.

What would the conversation look like?

"When I dare to be powerful, to use my strength in the service of my vision, then it becomes less and less important whether I am afraid."

– Audre Lorde

When the sexual door opens, it is a great time for the truth to come out. During these conversations, a vulnerable part of yourself gets to meet a vulnerable part of them. Generally, when it is someone you care about, there is an instinct to protect.

Several recommendations:

#1: **BREATHE!** Use of Tonglin (see p. 114) is wonderful in these situations. Breathe in anxiety, nervousness, and judgment and breathe out safety, security, and calm. Repeating this with a few deep breaths steadies nerves and allows for the commitment to be the best you can be in the conversation.

#2: **BE PRESENT.** Be conscious of the present moment as you are sharing your desire to be loved and innermost fear of rejection. It is better to focus on your words than wandering to how they may respond, what your partner is thinking, what this conversation implies, or what you will do tomorrow. By placing your awareness in this moment and giving attention, you could bear witness to a great transformation within yourself.

#3: **BE ACCOUNTABLE.** This is a willingness to answer for the outcomes of your choices, actions, and behaviors. Account for the fact that you created your entire world and this situation. When you are personally accountable, you stop assigning blame, making excuses, and "shoulda coulda woulda" on others. Take the fall when your choices cause problems; being a victim to your past does not allow for emotional growth.

#4: **BE CLEAR.** Know what you are going to do with that knowledge. Be clear and express yourself as unambiguously as possible. The clarity layer is where we can influence others. The words may not come easily, and your confidant may be hanging off a wire waiting, but that is okay! You can set the tone of the conversation with your verbal and nonverbal language, and they will respond in like. For instance, presenting herpes in a factual confident manner as a manageable virus will be perceived differently than presenting herpes as a shameful, embarrassing virus.

In uncertainty, I have started conversations with, "I want to talk to you about something important. I don't really know how to say this, but I am just going to say it the best I can because I want to put it out there." I have been met with a positive shift in the air of patience and time for me to figure out what I wanted to convey, which allowed for a more productive conversation.

Please be aware of your body's response as an important component of an emotional reaction. Not every move has a meaning, but your body language can also convey how you feel.

Eyes down, covered face: Guilt, self-condemnation, shame.

Excessively jerky movements: frustration, irritation.

Looking down or away: annoyance, frustration.

Talking with hand gestures or playing with jewelry: nervousness, anxiety, embarrassment.

Shrinking or Slumping: depression, despair, low spirits.

Still limbs, head up, steady speed of speech, eyes directed at the person you are speaking with: Confidence!

#4: **BE POWERFUL.** Power is the capability to influence others and your surroundings. This is a potent moment to express and realize your worth, knowing that you can be loved and that you love yourself. Everybody has the ability to be 100% powerful in our lives. We can choose to give that power away, but that is a conscious choice. Power can seldom work without an action, so go for it and be brave!

#5: **RESPOND, DO NOT REACT**: While these word choices may look like word semantics, in the reactive mode, the brain expresses fear and anger. There may be defensive positions where feelings of abandonment, worthlessness, loneliness or greed present. Reacting is instinctual, while responding is a conscious choice. In the responsive mode, the brain is calm, happy, and healthy but inquisitive. This stance stimulates thoughtful, compassionate conversation in a mature way. If someone behaves badly, it is not up to us to try and get them to behave.

This mindfulness may be best expressed by this example: a patient goes to the doctor for medication and returns for a follow-up visit. In one case, the doctor says you are *reacting* to a medication; in the other case, the doctor says you are *responding* to the medication. This fine line difference hones self-awareness.

"Though no one can go back and make a brand new start, anyone can start from now and make a brand new ending."

— Carl Bard

I don't even know where to begin; what should I say?

Feel free to rehearse this to commit it to memory, write it down to recite in front of them, record it on your phone to play in front of your partner. These suggestions will help until you find your own words to express what you would like.

Script Suggestion #1 for informing a new partner of your existing herpes diagnosis:

I have something to tell you because I think our relationship is heading in the direction of intimacy. Before we become sexually active, I want to tell you that I do have a diagnosis of herpes. I've had it for x long, and I am currently on treatment, or, I take treatment when I have an outbreak, or, I am on suppression. I think this is important for you to know so that you have a choice. If this isn't something you would like to continue, I understand. I'm saddened because I really like you, but this is where I'm at.

Script Suggestion #2 for a partner you have been with previously and you have recently been diagnosed with herpes:

I went to the doctor because I noticed an ulceration. The doctor is doing a culture and has a suspicion that it is herpes. I am currently on medication. It's important when I have this outbreak that we aren't sexually active because it is sexually transmitted. We can look on appropriate websites together. The doctor doesn't know which partner I got it from so I'm not saying that it's coming from you; it's just that I have the diagnosis now and I want to tell you.

Script Suggestion #3 for a partner whom you have been sexually active with and you have a known history of herpes:

I realize that we have been intimate, and I should have told you before but I was ashamed and scared. I don't want to be ashamed and scared anymore. I want to be very honest. I have herpes. We have not been active when I've had an outbreak. I understand if you are shocked and disappointed. I hope that we can move forward from this together.

What if they leave me? How do I handle rejection?

I would like to take a moment and congratulate you on choosing a higher expression of yourself! Applause for you for taking the first super scary step! Rejection can be despicable, but this can also be an incredible opportunity for growth. Perhaps this partner was too small to fit in your big story. This a great position for advancement by shifting perspective and focusing on yourself, your self-love, and your self-worth. From these experiences, a shiny version of yourself can emerge, filtering those who will be a contributor in your life and those who will detract from it.

When a future partner comes into our lives, we do not know anything about their past. They could have been a "good" person. They could have been a "bad" person. They could have been a cheater. They could have hidden their own STI history from us. All we know about a future partner is how they present now. In my case, I admit being dishonest and careless with other people's health, but I do not believe this makes me a "bad" person. I have grown from my past as I worked myself away from a punished position, and I appreciate that consideration as I move forward.

Do I need to have only one partner for the rest of my life?

No, absolutely not. In fact, you could have multiple partners at the same time if you wanted to. I am not promoting promiscuity, but you can practice safe sex as long as your partners are aware of the risk of herpes and appropriate protection is used. Enjoy your sex life—life is short!

What if I have given it to them, what do I tell them?

I would have hoped that if an outbreak on the other person occurred, it was because you had already told them. If they had come to you after you had told them and said, "I have an outbreak," I would recommend that they go to their physician to confirm with a culture and to start medication.

If it is a situation where you had not told the partner yet and they did have a positive culture and an outbreak, it is best at that point to choose. It may not have the best outcome but come clean and say, "I have herpes, and I know I wasn't honest with you." If they are angry, they have the right to be angry, and hopefully together you can move forward from the experience.

Are there any legal implications to herpes if I don't tell my partner?

There are no legal implications if someone was not informed of having sex with a herpes positive person. In California, HIV is the only actionable STI where there can be liability.

Please keep in mind that you may not know if your partner is being fully honest with you. Even in long term, monogamous relationships, we may not know based off of where the other person is in their honesty about their sexual history.

What happened when you told your partners?

When I finished writing this book and was preparing for publishing, I notified partners that I had been intimate with, remain in contact with as friends or acquaintances, and had not told my diagnosis before. Personally informing them before the book was released was important to me—for my own growth and out of respect. Below you will find my conversations and their messages to me. In Chapter 7, The Case Studies, you will see further development of Ben and Dan's perspective, the men I had spoken about at the beginning of this book.

I share my parade of partners to illustrate two things: these men have their own honest reactions: some supportive of me and some cluttered with their own issues with me. I respect all of them for their sincere and fair responses as I created these situations by hiding the truth from them. Second, I reveal my experiences to show that I still may not disclose well. I could not have predicted how my information will be received, and it is not my place to determine that for them.

Brett was the first boyfriend I had after I acquired HSV 1 in college. Brett and I dated for 2.5 years approximately 12 years ago. When it came time for him to move from New York to California after my first year of medical school, I freaked out and ended the relationship, conducting myself poorly. Out of the forgiveness in his heart and his persistence to maintain a friendship, we catch up perhaps once or twice a year via Facebook or in person. It was out of the blue that I contacted him, but not so strange that he would hear from me. Even after writing this book, I felt the pounding in my heart as I prepared what I would say.

I took a deep breath in and informed him: "I am calling because I am writing a book and I wanted you to know about it first. It is a book I believe will be impactful in the community. You see, I contracted herpes when I was 20 years old from a previous boyfriend. You and I dated after that, and I hid it from you. You know I have been doing emotional work with a life coach, and concealing this was inappropriate. I would like to believe that we were not sexually active when I had a lesion, but I honestly cannot remember that far to tell you 100%. I am sorry for hiding this from you; I hope you can forgive me." As I paused, I could hear Brett processing and taking breaths. Slowly, he articulated, "Thank you for letting me know. I know that must have been very hard for you. I am glad to hear this from you than from somewhere else. I haven't had an outbreak genitally ever in the past ... So ... Tell me, what more is your book about?" I was able to answer his questions and concerns, mostly about testing, what the lesions would look like, what this meant for his current girlfriend and children. After 30 minutes, Brett seemed reassured by our conversation, and he seamlessly transitioned the conversation to our current lives in terms of my recent job move, his children, and work. Our conversation ended with audible smiles over the phone and from him, "Thank you for being honest and telling me. It was great to hear from you and catch up."

This message is from Patrick, the partner who gave me herpes in college:

Hi Sheila,

Thanks for the note and congratulations on the book! I appreciate the heads up.

Some of my deepest and most heartfelt regrets center on how I conducted myself during our relationship. Hopefully I have matured into a better person.

Regarding the infection, feel free to write whatever you wish. You don't have to share it with beforehand. If there are passages that aren't particularly flattering then, well, I'm sure I deserve it. I can remember how surprised I was when you were diagnosed. I can still hardly believe it. I am so sorry.

I hope you and your family are doing well.

Good luck with the book!

Below are from other partners (forgive the grammar, English is their second language)

6/2, 12:03am

wow...lol....that was long - so far im good - so dont need to be worry - also i know alot about herpes and stds - its a pretty common thing , and not a big deal as long as u take care of it - but thank u for letting me know , i appreciate it ☺
wish u a good day and good health Xoxo

Hi Sheila
First I want to tell you that I forgive you. Our life was not easy because we live long way from each other and we had an impossible love. Don't be afraid of the way you treated me because i think it's normal. We had our own life. I'm happy because we broke together in good terms. I have a lot of questions about your new job, your book and what you said about herpes. I want to tell you lot of things about my sentimental life, my sexual life, about my family and my job. I think you didn't give me herpes but I'm not sure.

In this one, you can see my dear friend processing how he feels about the situation. I was writing him back before work:

6/1/16, 22:37:39: ■■■■: So what are you saying exactly
6/2/16, 06:03:34: Sheila Loanzon: Hey, Just woke up. I am saying that I had herpes and I didn't tell you. You may have already had it from someone before or after me and not known. If you haven't had an outbreak at this point then you probably didn't get it
6/2/16, 06:12:52: ■■■■: I didn't have an outbreak
6/2/16, 06:12:55: ■■■■: Thank God
6/2/16, 06:13:18: ■■■■: And we only had unprotected sex once right?
6/2/16, 06:13:34: ■■■■: But to be honest sheila.. its kinda f---ked up you didnt tell
6/2/16, 06:14:31: ■■■■: Well no outbreak for as far is i know. ☺
6/2/16, 06:15:05: Sheila Loanzon: Truthfully I don't remember if or how many times we had unprotected sex
I know it's f---ked up. I am very sorry and if I could take the situation back and be honest I would
6/2/16, 06:15:31: ■■■■: Yes but you can't..
6/2/16, 06:16:17: ■■■■: So probably i dont, have it
6/2/16, 06:16:48: Sheila Loanzon: If you haven't had anything this far you probably don't have it
6/2/16, 06:16:50: ■■■■: But.. its pretty messed up..
6/2/16, 06:17:02: Sheila Loanzon: I hope you can forgive me and we can be friends
6/2/16, 06:17:26: ■■■■: And i know i was there also so i could have said we should have used a condom but.. okay

6/2/16, 06:17:47: ██████████ : Well it feels like i got betrayed *is that the right word?*

6/2/16, 06:19:33: ██████████ : I'm not really sure what to think about this situation.. because thing is you knew! You knew it when we had sex and didn't tell.. that i do not like..

6/2/16, 06:19:43: ██████████ : If you didnt know and now you do and tell me that's a whole different scenario

6/2/16, 06:19:53: ██████████ : But you knew it all a long..

6/2/16, 06:19:56: ██████████ :

6/2/16, 06:20:43: ██████████ : And you're a doctor! In that specific erea also ☺

6/2/16, 06:21:04: ██████████ : You should have known better sheila..

6/2/16, 06:21:23: ██████████ : And i should not have been that naïeve

6/2/16, 06:21:37: ██████████ : I'm not angry

6/2/16, 06:21:51: ██████████ : I'm dissappointed

6/2/16, 06:22:53: ██████████ : Its just not cool

6/2/16, 06:23:12: ██████████ : But okay.. i probably dont have it.. since i never had an 'outbreak'

6/2/16, 06:23:52: Sheila Loanzon: I am somewhat reassured you don't have it. I am sorry ██████

6/2/16, 06:24:19: ██████████ : I cant say its okay but.. okay

6/2/16, 06:24:43: ██████████ : Thank God it isnt Hiv

6/2/16, 06:27:36: ██████████ : Okay..

6/2/16, 06:27:49: ██████████ : Hope it sells well

6/2/16, 06:27:53: ██████████ : Good luck with that

6/2/16, 06:28:11: ██████████ : You should give out free condoms with the book..

6/2/16, 06:29:13: ██████████ : I'm such an entrepreneur

6/2/16, 06:29:15: ██████████ : ☺

6/2/16, 06:29:45: Sheila Loanzon: You are!!! Good call!! I like both of these options, they would def give a unique spin. Getting a rec from a condom Corp would be way cool

6/2/16, 06:29:48: ██████████ : I Will be okay with 10% of the salesmargin

6/2/16, 06:30:37: Sheila Loanzon: K I really have to get into the shower and dressed

6/2/16, 06:30:40: Sheila Loanzon: I'm gonna be late

6/2/16, 06:30:43: ██████████ : Yeah sure no problem

6/2/16, 06:30:45: ██████████ : Ttyl

6/2/16, 06:30:50: ██████████ : If my d--k doesnt fall off

6/2/16, 06:30:57: ██████████ : ☺ ☺

6/2/16, 06:31:10: Sheila Loanzon: It won't. I promise your prized possession will stay attached

6/2/16, 06:31:19: ██████████ : ☺

Lastly, I received this response. This person and I had a tumultuous relationship and I have kept my distance until I reached out to him now. I agree that sending an email may not have been the most appropriate however you can see how varied the responses can be.

Sheila, your message was the first thing I woke up to today. With that being said, I must tell you, I am extremely disappointed in the way you handled this. (That's putting it politely.) I should not have to explain this to a grown adult, but the proper way to handle something like this would be to reach and out say, ██████████ I know it's been a while, but I'd really like to chat with you sometime and catch up. I've misplaced your number. Would you mind sending it to me again please? Or just text me at ......" You don't just launch a bloody missile through Facebook at someone telling them something like that. I'm actually shocked at the way you went about this.

I would have been happy to call you (an offer I have made in the not so distant past by the way, only to have ignored by you, just FYI).

All else I can say is that I guess I look forward to reading your book. Health wise, I am find. No issues. Luck of the draw I guess. If you reach out to anyone else, just FYI, get their contact info and speak to them. Do not drop shit like this on Facebook. So bad.

I woke up that morning and received the above messages. Honestly, I was relieved with some of the responses and disappointed in myself with the last one. I spoke to Dan about it that morning and in a succinct text, he pinpointed how we can all view life.

██████████████████ Baba don't worry about the past...what's done is done and nothing can be changed. You can try to make amends but it's not always possible. I love you in the here and now that's what matters!!

Chapter Eight

STORIES IN AND OUT OF THE
EXAM ROOM

*"Life's challenges are not supposed to paralyze you. They're supposed
to help you discover who you are."*

— Bernice Johnson Reagon

*All names and identifying details have been changed or omitted
to protect the privacy of individuals.*

Sarah was a 32-year-old patient who came in for her first
prenatal visit. Reviewing her history in the electronic medical
record, I reviewed her diagnosis of herpes. While she had a hard
time meeting my eye and kept shifting in her seat, she made
it very clear she did not want anyone in her family to know,
including her husband. I reassured her that with HIPAA[44] her
information was well protected and, therefore, confidential. I
updated the chart specifically stating her desire to withhold this
information from the family in the problem list and through
our office visit note. I did inform her that while it was written
on her chart this was confidential, sometimes information
inadvertently is revealed. I acknowledged that she did not want
to tell her partner, supported her in that decision, and reminded
her that she will need Acyclovir suppression starting at 36 weeks,

---

[44] acronym for the Health Insurance Portability and Accountability Act that was
passed by Congress in 1996. HIPAA establishes national standards to protect individuals' medical records and other personal health information. The Rule requires
appropriate safeguards to protect the privacy of personal health information, and
sets limits and conditions on the uses and disclosures without patient authorization.

then told her to let me know if she has any outbreaks. I also notified her that if she had any symptoms that she may need a primary cesarean delivery to prevent any harm to her baby. The diagnosis remained concealed throughout the pregnancy and labor, and her baby was born without issues.

Ariana is a 31-year-old patient who repeatedly came to my office with symptoms of vaginal discharge. One day she came in with painful ulcerations, which I confirmed was herpes. Because Ariana came in so frequently, I got to know her and through her, her partner. He worked often so they were only together on the weekends. Ariana had difficulty understanding where she got her outbreak and found that he was in denial himself. She would point out where he would have outbreaks and inform him she did not want to be sexually active. He called her silly and refused to see his physician. She felt that her ob-gyn was the only one who could give her appropriate information. She would doubt herself, come in crying and helpless, and call herself "stupid" because she thought he was right.

While Ariana did have other social issues going on, she came to my office due to significant cocaine drug abuse. We got her the appropriate care that she needed, and three months later, she came in to see me. She had since left that partner due to the realization she was in a verbally abusive relationship. Beaming, she declared she was no longer emotionally crippled and was strong enough to survive on her own. She was grateful for the experience because she hit the very bottom and then fought within herself to climb out to the brighter side.

Joie, a 31 year old whom I originally worked with in the hospital, became a close friend of mine and subsequently my patient. She had been in a tumultuous long-term relationship with Reggie, during which she received chlamydia, genital warts, and lastly, herpes. Her chief complaint was a 3-day history of a vaginal irritation with unbearable pain when walking and when urine would hit the side wall of her vagina.

I took a viral culture of the sores and confirmed the diagnosis a day later. On the phone call giving her the diagnosis, she was very stoic and accepted her diagnosis quietly. She tells me now in hindsight as I write this book that she was crying when she went home. She felt dirty and betrayed. She thought to herself "Who is going to love me now? Should I blame myself or blame him? I'm strong but how am I going to get through this?"

Reggie adamantly denied the infection came from him and wanted to emphasize he was not with other people. Joie felt confused at the time and stated that while it took some time, she knew the only way to survive was to confide in strong, educated women. She surrounded herself with a chosen group of support such as myself, which she felt housed sensitivity and knowledge and her best girlfriends who were open, accepting, and reassured her. Joie attributes this community of safety as helping her through this change in her health.

During the first year of her diagnosis, Joie had outbreaks every month. She started daily suppression medication for her own sanity and to prevent spreading the infection. A pattern emerged: when she was stressed out (brother unexpectedly passing away, work and school stress), she would have an outbreak.

After recovering from her break up with Reggie, Joie was very careful when choosing sexual partners and religious using protection. She eventually met someone special one year later through online dating. She knew she was going to have to be honest about her diagnosis to explain the use condoms on a regular basis. Jason was open and accepting as Joie divulged her full STI history. Without reservation, he loved her and they became engaged a year later.

Several times when Joie initiated intimacy, Jason pushed her away, saying he had a headache. She confronted him gently asking him, "Is it because you have an outbreak?" Jason replied quietly, "Yes." Joie urged him, "Please let me know when this happens. I want to be your partner in this. I feel guilty, and I see that you are on your phone reading about it and watching educational videos. I am here." Jason has started suppression medication and never blamed or shamed her. They married last month and plan to start a family soon.

Laura is a 55-year-old psychiatrist who enjoyed the sexual freedoms of the '70s and '80s. For nearly 20 years, she had periodic vaginal fissures that she attributed to jean seams rubbing. When an outbreak coincided with her annual pap exam, she asked if the small cuts were anything concerning. She was shocked that the sores were herpes and immediately burst into tears. Her main concern was telling her husband, and she cried all the way home, wondering if he would think she cheated. She was greatly relieved when he calmly heard her news and reassured her that it was nothing that would change how he felt about her and their marriage. It was quickly a non-issue for them. He has not contracted herpes. They continue to have a strong, active sex life.

Martha and Alan, a young couple, were virginal when they met. They got married, and during their marriage, he cheated on her. Alan was honest with her from the beginning, and he also admitted from this extramarital indiscretion he got herpes. Martha contracted the virus and while she was seeing a psychologist for one year with the hope to move past this event, she had difficulty moving on because her frequent outbreaks were a constant reminder of the infidelity. "I did everything right! I was a virgin, I got married, and here I am being punished. Why do I have to suffer from something I never did?" They are still choosing to be together because of their religion, despite the cold relationship that remains.

Shannon, a 37-year-old woman and patient, came into the office for a routine postpartum visit after she delivered her second baby. When I first met her and her husband at her first prenatal visit of her first pregnancy, I was struck with how comfortable and open she was when I reviewed her medical history in front of her husband. There was no uncomfortable silence or shifting of her eyes when I informed her how her herpes diagnosis would affect her pregnancy. I had not been fully open at that time, and I admired her confidence.

I saw her after I decided to write this book and asked her to share her story. Shannon admitted that she has only had two partners in her life and recounted that she was with her high school boyfriend whom she had married and found out he had cheated on her during their marriage. She had sparse outbreaks in college but confidently moved forward with her life. She met her husband and immediately informed him of having herpes. She admits, "I found I was harder on myself than my partner was." Jose loved her exactly as she was and did not bat an eyelash regarding moving forward together. They now have two healthy beautiful children together, and Shannon considers herself blessed and fully loved.

Ben, the same guy I dated at the beginning of my story, proofread my book and adds (I copied his emailed words verbatim):

"When you and I had the conversation, my attitude was, 'I may marry this woman. She's obviously upset, how can I be honest with my own concern but support her when she feels so vulnerable'."

"After we had our conversation I really wanted to talk to somebody. Any friend who could understand and hold my hand. I was really conscious that somebody might gossip or put two and two together and know more about you than I wanted."

I was reminded of the old Jewish prohibition on gossip. One lady who used to gossip felt bad and went to the rabbi (teacher). She asked if there was anything she could do. The rabbi thought about and told her to get a big bed pillow, and stab it in her backyard with a knife. "Then scatter the feathers around and come talk to me again." The lady thought he was crazy, but did as he said. Rabbis are supposed to be wise! When she came back he told her, "Now, gather up all the feathers!" "But that's impossible! I scattered them like you told me, and now the wind has taken them everywhere!" "And that, ma'am is the problem with gossip."

Eventually, I found a very sex-positive couple, who greatly reassured me that herpes is really no more than an annoying rash—one that got unreasonably stigmatized as drug companies went looking for clients—and that I should get tested and worry about the relationship, rather than anything else."

Dan, my current partner, and I were discussing my book and I asked if he had any outbreaks since we had been together. He admitted that he had not. I asked if my disclosure surprised him. He gently informed me, "I had a past partner who admitted she had herpes, too, so when you told me, I didn't think it was a big deal. I had read about it when I was with her and found out a lot of people had it. It didn't matter to me. I really liked you then and love you now." In our relationship, we open heartedly choose each other as partners. We have welcomed difficult conversations as a way to deepen our connection and grow together. This type of devotion is so magical and evolves us both!

Chapter Nine

INTRODUCTION TO SELF-HELP PORTION

YOU MAY HAVE noticed when you decided to choose this book that the initials after my name are D.O. and not M.D. D.O. stands for Doctor of Osteopathy. In the US, there are two types of separate, but equal, medical schools: Allopathic (M.D.) and Osteopathic (D.O.). Allopathic and osteopathic medical schools have the same undergraduate requirements and require the same entrance testing (MCAT). Both are four years and require the same series of medical board examinations. Osteopathic medical school appealed to me because it combines the focus of symptom-based approaches with the holistic perception of medicine, offering great versatility. Osteopaths are doctors first. Beyond that categorization, however, osteopaths are armed with knowledge gained through significant hours spent learning manipulative techniques. For residency, though, I chose an allopathic program based on the excellent medical and surgical training offered. I do not practice osteopathic manipulative medicine currently; however, the ability to diagnose with my hands through medical school and residency training is useful every day.

I bring this aspect of my education to you because one of the basic tenets of Osteopathy is *"structure affects function"*. One of my favorite examples of how osteopathy can work is a young child who consistently gets ear infections. An osteopath can obtain a history and evaluate the patient (not unlike an M.D.) and discover that when the baby was born, the mother

98 • YES, I HAVE HERPES

had a prolonged delivery with pushing over three hours that subsequently resulted in a vacuum delivery. This external large force on the fetal head caused some distortions in the fetal skull bones and thus does not allow for appropriate drainage of ear fluid once the baby was born. This can lead to chronic ear infections. Through a series of manipulative techniques over a period of time, the D.O. can perform cranial work on the baby where dysfunction exists and coax the bones into correct position, allowing for appropriate drainage and hopefully decrease infection in the future.

Just as in this situation where structural bones affect functional drainage, I also believe that structure in our lives can affect the way we function in life. I bring these tools to you as they worked for me to give structural guidelines to slowly envelope me in self-love to function wholly in my community. There are many tools out there; however, these specific worked for me and I invite you to use them with me.

SHEILA'S SELF-LOVE BOOTCAMP

One of the major beliefs I previously held was the need for external validation to justify my internal worth. However, the approval I desired is best generated within, rather than from outside sources (partners, friends, financial gains). These projects given to me by Julien over time gave me tools to confidently stand on my own and strength to move away from the condemnation I would put myself through. Better mental health is associated with higher self-esteem, less loneliness, and less internalized feelings. It can be difficult to foster positive identities. Herpes can manifest feelings of shame, denial, avoidance, hate of self, envy for those who do not have herpes, and distorted negative self-body image. Lowered self-esteem, depression, hopelessness, and pessimism are fostered. Internalized phobia to herpes is common due to these feelings.

Through these tips, I invite you to let your light shine through again. I am here to support you.

LIST OF 200

When I started my conscious work with Julien, my mind was rattled with constant beratement: I don't feel smart enough. I don't feel pretty enough. Why don't I have a loving partner yet? Why don't I look like my friends? Redirection occurred when I was instructed to create a list of 200 qualities that are unique, interesting, and different about me. This powerful tool can be used to boost self-worth and confidence.

I found the first 75 to be easy! To share a few examples: Generous, witty, I look young for my age, I have great teeth and bright smile, I am well liked by patients, excellent surgical skills, I speak Spanish, I have a great family, I can make friends easily, organized, excellent at multitasking, etc. Once I hit 125, it became more difficult; but I was proud of the list I had created because I realized I am so much more unique and special than I acknowledged. Often, I would read it before I went to bed and something magical happened ...

#169: I have herpes. WOW! What a huge pivotal moment!!! This was the moment a traumatic life event I had been evading transformed me into a more unique and special person. Tears were in my eyes when I wrote it down, and I stared at that spot on my spreadsheet for several minutes, feeling so proud of the accomplishment.

I encourage you to create a list of your own and reflect on it when a boost of confidence is needed. The characteristic that you despise, consider mundane, or judge yourself for may be a unique aspect of yourself wrapped in one package. I looked at my list when I started writing this book. My list is now at 227 and grows time to time—how far can your list go?

I FEEL LOVED WHEN...

A theory Julien had was I sought relationships to fill a void of love that I was seeking, mainly in a partner. This was the reason I immediately jumped into relationships and ignored some telltale red flags. In conjunction with building my self-confidence, simultaneously with the List of 200, this exercise was to list the beautiful experiences when I feel loved.

My list starts out: "I feel loved when...

I am appreciated.
I am valued for who I am.
Someone gives me a warm hug.
When a friend sits with me while I'm crying uncontrollably.
Someone invites me to lunch.
I have a good friend in front of me."

My list continued in this fashion and included gestures from my friends and family. As I reached #40, I decided to broaden my list to my environment. Witnessing a child being kissed by a parent, a kind deed done for someone else, a beautiful sunrise, and the sun warming my skin invokes the same "warm feelings all over."

It was on a gorgeous spring morning when I was driving to work when the lightbulb clicked in my head like a smack on my forehead: "Oh. My. God!!! There is love ALL around me! I AM a loved person. I was created a loved person. I live in a world with loved people and people who love me. I exude it and now I truly feel it!" I sobbed in my car for five minutes after that revelation. What a wonderful joy to feel love from all around you and within yourself!

I encourage you to create a list of when you feel loved. Make it juicy and clear and I hope you have the same head-smacking reaction at some point that I had!

6 WAYS TO LOVE YOURSELF: HOW TO MOVE FORWARD WITH CONFIDENCE AND SELF-LOVE

1. Shift Your Perspective

I am SO worth it. I think it is important for women to take time for themselves. I find in my practice that women spend so much time managing and facilitating for their husbands, their children, and significant others. Women have a tendency to really put themselves on the back burner to sacrifice for others in their lives. It is not uncommon for me to see women in their 40s and 50s who are exhausted, depressed, anxious, and have not made themselves a priority and have forgotten how to take care of themselves.

I encourage something restorative and make yourself the focal point: take a walk outside and breathe fresh air, read something inspiring, take a nap. Shifting from an empty gas tank to a full gas tank gives energy and strength and can lighten our emotional load. I find when I take better care of myself, I can take better care of others. This can be likened to being in an airplane and the oxygen mask drops due to altitude changes. The instructions given by the flight attendants on the plane are to "place an oxygen mask on yourself, and then place it on others." If we are without oxygen, what good can we be to others? Taking time for yourself means you are cared for and ultimately signifies you are worth it. The universe and others will respect that. Self-care is like a piggy bank—you cannot keep withdrawing without depositing. You will ultimately find yourself emotionally withdrawn and bankrupt.

My experience: This took some time for me to learn because I am, at my core, a people pleaser. I would bend over backwards for patients, friends, and family, doing what was expected of me, yet not doing what was best for me in the long run. I was exhausted, burned out, and financially overwhelmed until I realized that it is not my responsibility to take care of them.

By managing others, I was expending my own energy, which could have been spent taking care of myself.

I started clearing one hour a day after work to take a Pilates or boxing class. I took up mosaics, adult coloring books, and party planning and discovered my creative side felt nurtured with the beautiful colors, organizing, plotting, and choosing how to showcase a beautiful design and my aesthetic dreams. I found myself happier and energetically charged. By being ego-centric for a small amount of time daily, I had an internal fountain of joy that I was freely open to sharing with others.

2. Trust Your Gut

This age-old advice is due to the instinctual method that we all have built into our bodies. I realize that this can be "hokey" to some people and most of my physician colleagues. However, imagine how powerful a method could be by reliably telling us what is best for us. This challenging system can be difficult to tap into; however, through a year-long process, I discovered my internal gut has never steered me wrong. My body gives me the answers I need; and the more I have used it, the more in tune it seems to be. If the answer I receive to my question seems odd or not in the favor I would like, I have realized there is a bigger picture I was not privy to seeing yet. I listed out all the times when I thought my gut had steered me wrong, and I discovered that it, in fact, directed me exactly where I needed to go.

When I succumbed to my gut and trusted it in big decisions, I no longer blamed or became angry when things did not seem to go my way. It removed that pressure and in turn, improved my outlook.

My experience: Gut instinct, gut wrenching, feeling in my gut... I had those instinctive intuitions, and I used to ignore them to get what (I thought) I wanted. I use my gut now to decide on a trip to a certain location, when to buy tickets, if I should go on a specific retreat, whether to text the guy I am dating, which job opportunity would best suit me. Using my gut saved time from the back and forth in my head and steered me in the right direction.

When dating online with multiple pursuers, I used my gut to determine if it was right to continue dating certain gentlemen. I followed my gut wholeheartedly, which I believe saved me from staying in relationships too long or dating men who were inappropriate for me. Guesswork on how they felt about me no longer existed. It came down to my gut informing me, and what was right for ME.

I also notice when I am facing a stressful situation or unbeknownst emotional stress, my gut feels twisted in knots, I feel nauseous, lose my appetite, or have loose stools. This is a physical manifestation of turmoil, and I encourage the readers to note how their body reacts when there is an emotional component to a situation.

3. Enjoy the process of life

"We are products of our past, but we don't have to be prisoners of it."
— Rick Warren, *The Purpose Driven Life: What on Earth Am I Here for?*

Trusting that life is always bringing you exactly what you need in divine time can be difficult to believe sometimes. However, having faith that the universe is always conspiring for everyone's greatest good is a wonderful way to move about life. Take time to slow down, savor the experience, and reflect. I am a huge supporter of celebrating accomplishments, no matter how small or large. Celebrating invites beauty, laughter, joy, playfulness, delicious food, and pleasuring company. This can build a magnetic community and excitement for life.

My experience: Being a Type A personality, a surgeon, and an overall go-getter kind of person, I found frustration in relationships that would not go my way. I put in the work and the effort and was a good person, why wasn't I getting what I wanted and deserved? The key component is that I have no control over the other person! I realize that all the situations that I was forcing were actually steering me in the wrong direction. Once I let go of the reins and trusted the universe/God, I had more raw joyous moments, found more compatible mates, and expended less energy spinning my wheels stressing over what I was not getting. I get to enjoy all the wonderful experiences I am receiving and live in the moment!

4. Face Your Demons

"Don't be afraid of new ideas. Be afraid of old ideas. They keep you where you are and stop you from growing and moving forward. Concentrate on where you want to go, not on what you fear."

— Anthony Robbins

Personally, I had an issue with intimacy ("Into Me You See"). My communication skills with colleagues, staff, and patients were extraordinary, and I could sext partners without problems, but I had difficulty being intimate and expressing my feelings. Instead of getting bigger and leaning into an experience, I would burrow into a hole, not understanding my feelings and slinking away. Luckily, Julien provided a safe space and time without pressure for me to investigate what I was feeling. Nobody can blame you for having an emotion because you feel what you feel. I wanted to dig into my life and my deep rooted issues and break free.

Take the time to deal with your own history, make peace within yourself, find forgiveness, learn to love others, and move on in a lighter sense. For a person who has been abused, ashamed, or abandoned, those are very difficult things to deal with, but they make you who you are. In a victim role, we become unable to take any ownership and thus grow. I encourage you to find the source of your pressures–family, media, politics, etc. Clearing the things that dragged me down opened room for positive uplifting things to happen for me, and suddenly the "evil" things in my life did not outweigh the great in my life.

My experience: I grew up in a predominantly Caucasian Catholic culture as my immigrated Filipino parents encouraged me to assimilate in. I followed the current fads, became the 4.0 GPA cheerleading captain, dated a football player, and wanted to fit in. I even dyed my hair blonde and put in blue contacts. Joking with my good friend, Sanaz, we postulated we were Caucasian for a good portion of our lives until filling out college applications and we had to bubble in our ethnic backgrounds.

My parents valued education tremendously, and pressure to become successful as a doctor, lawyer, or engineer in the United States was highly regarded. I had visions of becoming a doctor (it sounded great to say, I was compassionate and kind, and I had excellent grades to support it), but when I was 20 years old, my father passed away from brain cancer in 9 months, and the idea was solidified.

High school came fairly easily to me. Although in college I received several science awards, I toiled day and night to earn my grades. Standardized testing was difficult for me; however, my MCAT scores gained me a spot in medical school. Step 1 USMLE exams are done the second year of medical school and objectively test knowledge on chemistry, biology, and reading comprehension, not medical knowledge practiced on a daily basis. I crumbled when I received my scores and did not pass by *one* point. I repeated the exam and soared through Step 1 and subsequently Step 2 in my fourth year of med school, and Step 3 was done after my intern year of residency.

My life has been about overcoming obstacles. Our goals do not falter easily. I had to fight for the things that I value; nothing was handed to me easily. All of these tribulations could have reinforced that I was not good enough. These experiences could have proven lacking self-worth. Reflecting back, these situations were, in fact, building my strength up for the career and opportunities that I see ahead of me.

I lost my father at a young impressionable age. I did not have a strong male role model and began looking for that in the men that I was dating. Through arduous internal work, I realized my own self-worth and gained independence from the cultural norm that I *had* to be partnered with someone.

In my career, creatively tackling difficult concepts is joyful for me. I had to find ways in medical school and residency to understand the basic principles myself. I believe patients understand their bodies better due to the way I explain medical concepts to them. For instance, topics such as hormones, polycystic ovaries, birth control, and labor all of a sudden make sense. I have overheard my examples and explanations in conversations with patients from other clinicians in my office. I could have identified as the person who did not pass Step 1 by one point; however, I choose that to be the moment I learned to push myself further.

5. Surrender

Trust in a bigger picture and know that there is a larger lesson that we do not yet see. A larger power does love you, even though you may not see it, and it does not help to fight it. I found that things go smoothly when I allow things to happen, rather than trying to make things happen.

My experience: Recently I went on a yoga retreat with a group of ten women in their late 20s to late 30s. We had known each other as acquaintances from our studio, but some had been close friends for many years. I arrived separately from the group and was told the wrong time for the welcome dinner. I arrived to the restaurant one hour later than the rest. I felt somewhat insecure and out of place since they had already "self-ied" and toasted the celebration. Throughout the three-day retreat, I felt a high school type uneasiness and anxiety as I did my best to fit with these tall gorgeous blonde beauties. I laughed at their jokes, I walked up to the group and attempted to join in conversations, and I attempted to surround myself around them at the pool.

After completing beach yoga one morning, we took a celebratory photo and I found myself in the middle of the group. Due to shadowing, position of the sun, and my dark complexion, all you could see was my white teeth smiling in the photo. It was hysterical to everyone else but a deep cut inside me. I felt sunken into the middle of the group shadowed by women around me. I turned away brushing tears from my eyes as these women giggled, not at me of course, for they did not know the scarring that existed.

I had an inkling I was not acting like my confident self which was causing frustration. Instead of joining the afternoon workout, I took the afternoon for myself to figure out what was going on. I sat by the beach, did some meditation and deep breathing, and kept asking, "Why do I want to fit in? Why do I want to fit in?" It dawned on me. I was *trying to fit in*? I was the only Asian woman in this group of 10 blondes and I was trying fit in? With tears in my eyes I realized I was created unique and special exactly as I am. Why be another blond in this group when I could stand individually and be exactly as I was lovingly created.

At that moment, I felt relief and love for myself. It was as if chains had been broken free. On that sandy beach amongst the waves, I decided to write this book to celebrate my incomparable self. Ironically, the following two days when I did not overly exert myself to fit in and surrendered to the experience, the blondes showed a larger interest in me and wanted to sit next to me for a change.

6. Surround yourself with a loving community

I have discovered in life that sometimes we need to lean on friends and family to pull us out of our own condemnation and smack us on the head with reality.

My experience: I have been very fortunate to have a loving group of people around me, and it is in the comfort of their love that I was able to blossom. When I informed one my closest family friends I was writing this book, Tory's eyes got wide and I thought she was judging me and my herpes. However, once I finished telling her my story, she burst into tears and admitted she felt so saddened. She clarified further and stated, "It isn't because of what you think. I am so sad that you felt you had to go through this alone." Friends and family want to be there for us; we just have to let them.

5 WAYS TO IMPROVE YOUR SELF-WORTH

1. Look for support outside of yourself

There are many unifying coalitions fostering inclusiveness and interest to encourage awareness and acceptance. If you prefer to find a support group, there are many available publicly and privately websites using passwords to enter. I encourage patients to find those niches where you realize you are not alone.

My experience: Julien Adler[45] is an executive coach, a master hypnotherapist, a leadership trainer and is perfect for emotional alignment for me. The cultural pressures and the training I had before ended up being retrained because of his coaching. Look for self-help books; look for tips you can incorporate into your life. Things that used to take me six months to recover from now occur within three days. The things that used to frustrate me no longer exist because my coping mechanisms have changed. Through firm tools and support I have been able to respond

---

[45] www.julienadler.com

and navigate through life with ease which causes less turmoil, lack of sleep, and internal strife.

2. Look within

There are a broad variety of meditation techniques. They all self-regulate the mind in some way. You may not be great at quieting your mind in the beginning, but you will end up expanding your mind and finding answers you had not noticed before.

Meditation for beginners:

You can do two minutes of sitting a day, increasing it every few weeks or so. Some people like to meditate first thing in the morning, some at night. I recommend not getting caught up on how to do it, just sit and just do.

Start with noticing how you are feeling. Are you feeling anxious, busy, tired?

Count your breaths and take this chance to look inward. Breathe all the way through your nose and breathe out to the bottom of your lungs. If you lose focus, gently bring your mind back to your breath.

Wiggle your toes to notice your body and check in with yourself.

You can work with guided meditations, mantras, or listen to the ambient noises around. It is not always easy or peaceful because it can bring thoughts and emotions to the surface. Continue to sit and you will find an improvement in your self-worth just by taking this time for yourself.

> "Unlike a maze whose intent it is to get us lost, the labyrinth is designed to get us found."
>
> — Unknown

My experience: In 2014, I took myself to Bali for a yoga retreat. When I was there, my yoga instructor for the week took one look at me and said I would benefit from meditation. He could see thoughts ruminating in my head when I was supposed to be "quiet." He gave me mala beads and asked me to repeat "om tare tuttare ture soha" touching each bead. Even with this simple act, I found that my mind continued to be active in this seated position.

In 2015, I was at a juice fast retreat in Palm Desert doing a walking meditation through an ancient labyrinth. While wandering aimlessly between the rocks, various answers to questions I did not know existed flooded me. I walked the labyrinth daily and found new revelations each time. I have found that walking meditations help me the best, and I encourage you to find which meditation works the best for you.

3. Change the Subconscious

Hypnotherapy and psychotherapy can be used to create subconscious change in the form of new thoughts, attitudes, patterns, and feelings. We are programmed by previous actions, thoughts, experiences, and things we have learned from the outside world.

My experience: Julien incorporates a variety of techniques with his clients, including hypnotherapy. I am not sure the specifics of his work on me. However, the finesse and grace that I now have navigating through life and difficulties shows evidence of his skill. Previous upheld walls of fairy tale beliefs, ill-conceived cultural expectations, and familial pressures have vanished, and the construct that I live in is purely in my greatest interest. Because of this strong influence, I offer you a hypnotherapy track specific for herpes. Please refer to my website www.DrSheilaGYN.com for a free download.

4. Treat Yourself Well, Build Yourself Up

When you make yourself a priority, other people will treat you as a priority. This can be as simple as buying something new for yourself, doing your makeup, or doing your hair for the day. Treating yourself well is also being kind to yourself, utilizing positive affirmations, and eliminating negative self-talk. We can externally program ourselves to see our worth.

5. Purify Your Body

By detoxifying the body and pursuing restorative practices such as juice cleansing, massage, healthy eating, and exercise, you are caring for your temple and loving your body. Take a moment to absorb the nutrients of nature and consciously exercise. When we care for our body in this way, we are signaling to our subconscious that we are loved and we are worthy.

My experience: Most of my friends would describe me as being open to alternative treatments, and thus I have run the gamut of detoxification spas, juice fasts, and a multitude of spa treatments. The most recent one I did was called raindrop therapy, which helps treat viruses and bacteria. I did not learn the science behind it, but I have to admit that I felt relaxed and rejuvenated afterward. I believe that aspect was worth it.

SHEILA'S TRICKS: 5 WAYS TO COPE WITH STRESS (AND POSSIBLY AVOID HERPES BREAKOUTS)

"Everything can be taken from a man but one thing: the last of the human freedoms — to choose one's attitude in any given set of circumstances, to choose one's own way."

— Viktor E. Frankl, *Man's Search for Meaning*

1. Physical Activity

Exercise stimulates systems of the body that can assist in the process of detoxification, toning of muscles, increase oxygen intake for energy, and stimulate circulation for proper fueling and healing of tissue cells. New activity patterns can promote feelings of calm and wellbeing, while releasing endorphins[46] in the brain to energize spirits and improve how you feel. Exercise can also serve as a distraction, allowing quiet time to break the cycle of negative thoughts that feed depression and anxiety.

Many patients discuss their walking habits, and while I do appreciate the weight bearing exercise for women and their bones, it is important to incorporate cardiovascular activity for heart health. Similarly, I encourage women as we age to lift weights—I promise you will not bulk up like Arnold Schwarzenegger; you do not have the testosterone to build muscles like that! As we get older, we lose muscle mass, and lifting weights helps build and tone those muscles so it can burn calories when you are sleeping!

It is not uncommon for patients coming in for their routine gynecology exam to state they do not exercise due to a foot or knee injury. Your overall body is so much more than your one foot or knee! Find a way to make it work: swimming decreases gravitational pull, pilates can be done mostly on the back, lifting weights sitting in a chair- if no weights are available lift those heavy purses or cans of veggies. I started doing Pilates reformer because I had bunion surgery and would be non weight bearing for 3 months using crutches and walking boot. I found that laying on my back worked my core abdominal muscles and I built flexibility and strength in my arms while I decreased foot swelling with my feet placed in the air. No more excuses, you can find a way to work out!

My experience: When I was younger, I was a trained ballet dancer and transitioned into cheerleading in high school and college. After college, I lost that drive to exercise. 2014 was deemed my "Mind, Body, Spirit" year. I discovered my love for boxing (pink

---

[46] Endorphins: powerful neurotransmitters.

gloves, of course!) and Pilates (my childhood ballet dancing had a chance to come out again). Boxing offers cardiovascular aggressive release for me, and Pilates embodies deep breathing and stretching out the body and tension. Please find what works for you and move your body to get maximum stress relief. Once that stress releases outward instead of within yourself, your body is free to relax and breathe, as well. I generally encourage two to three days a week at first to avoid burnout and slowly work your times up if you have availability in your schedule.

2. Sleep

Sleep is so important for the recovery and restoration of your energy and mind. A good night's sleep keeps your heart healthy, prevents weight gain, boosts your immune system, prevents headaches, and can influence your sex life. Memory has a tendency to improve, and your body will repair faster. People who sleep less have a tendency to be anxious and more stressed.

It is not surprising that celebrity Jennifer Lopez looks stunning at 46 years old after following a strict diet and exercise regimen and claims, "I love a good 9 or 10 hours, but I can never get that. So 7 or 8 is mandatory. If I don't get it, I just don't feel right. I start to feel crazy, I get emotional, and I feel tired all the time." Cindy Crawford divulges at 48 years old, "If I look back over 24 years, for sure it starts with sleep."

Yes, perhaps for these models and celebrities the genetics they inherited and finances to afford top makeup artists and stylists play a role in their longevity. However, I suspect their focus to help themselves by treating their bodies well makes a large difference.

My experience: In my chosen profession, sleep can be difficult to come by for an obgyn. Babies are born in the middle of the night and surgical complications can occur in the 23rd hour of a 24-hour hospital call. I do make it a point after a 24-hour shift to take a nap for several hours and then go to bed at a decent hour that night. The emotions that arise from lack of sleep, such as frustration, anger, and irritation, luckily only last me a shift. However, if sleep is lacking, I find that emotions pull through the rest of my day.

3. Tonglen

This is a breathing and relaxation exercise based in Tibetan Buddhist traditions. It is a powerful tool in not only transforming ourselves in tense moments but also in impacting others.

Visualize expansion as you breathe in any negative thoughts, emotions, or energies around you. Transforming the energy, you then breathe out loving kindness, compassion, and healing.

See https://www.upaya.org/dox/Tonglen.pdf for more detail of the practice.

My experience: A few years ago I performed a hysterectomy on a young woman who sustained a surgical complication, a common complication with major surgeries. She required unforeseen hospitalization and additional surgeries. Her family was expecting her to return immediately to care for her ailing mother and when my patient was not improving as rapidly as he preferred, her father became irate, condescending, and irrational. He refused to be guided to a separate room and security had to be called as bystanders in the hallway while I discussed her case with him. As he began his sharply abusive attack of her care by myself and the hospital, I used his five minute monologue to do Tonglen breathing. I breathed in his anger, frustration, irritation, and helplessness as he ranted while methodically breathing out calm, understanding, and patience. I was amazed to find his rapid speech slowed, his voice lowered, his anger stance was replaced with stillness and in his piercing eyes I found fear and fatigue. We moved to a family quiet room and I shared his concerns and intent to improve his daughter's health. The conversation ended in prayer, his hands warmly grasping mine as we prayed for his daughter's speedy recovery.

4. Positive Self-Talk and Reframing Negative Thoughts

Positive reframe strategies take the "stress" out of stressors— when we reframe, we look at the same situation in a new way that highlights possibilities and gets us out of feeling trapped. Whether we realize it or not, when we are faced with a stressor, we have the ability to control our reaction to it. Some may say this is not possible! Stressors exist in the external world, and we have to react to it. However, if we changed how our mind reacts to these events, would they still be as stressful?

"I can't do this" → "I will do the best that I can."
"Everything is going wrong" →"I will take this one step at a time."
"I hate when this happens" → "You know how to deal with this, you have done it before."
"I must not be worthy"→ "I am worthy."
"I feel dirty" → "I won't let this problem get me down."
"I can't be loved again."→"I will find the one who loves me for who I am."

5. Write It Out

Moving worries from head to paper is a great stress reducer. Writing helps you think about events and removes you from the situations that made you angry, sad, or frustrated. This momentary forgetfulness causes your breathing to slow as you concentrate on words and stops the stress/worry cycles in our heads. Writing a stream of consciousness is similar to walking meditation.

My experience: when ruminating or angry at someone previously, sleepless nights would frustrate me. I would wake up at 3am not having released the emotions. I would begin looking for confrontations via text wars or angry phone calls. I could destroy dating relationships with my strong words and angry voice. By journaling, these automatic thoughts transferred emotions to a piece of paper—by the morning these emotions did not have the same intensity and I usually ended up tossing the paper away. It was not extensive expressive writing—jotting down a few bullet points or paragraphs (as if I was speaking to the person) protected my relationships and helped me keep my sanity!

Ho'oponopono, The Hawaiian Prayer

This is a traditional Hawaiian prayer that is very powerful and simple at the same time. In the Hawaiian Dictionary, "Ho'oponopono" is a "mental cleansing: family conferences in which relationships were set right through prayer, discussion, confession, repentance, and mutual restitution and forgiveness." This harmonizing practice is a way of nurturing the pain and suffering within. We can mother the children of our emotions so that we can generate more compassion. Simply, this practice makes right the relationship with myself through the psyche, subconscious and conscious mind, and experience of life.

Life is a duality of accepting and integrating the good and bad. When there is acceptance, the need for forgiveness or revenge disappears. We can choose the way we feel, and this is a powerful way of "making friends" with the parts of us that we resist and judge. Welcoming difficult things and thanking them for showing us the experience so we can grow is extremely powerful. We are choosing to elevate ourselves to the next soft, relaxed level. We are all part of the same reality; therefore, if we heal disharmony within ourselves, perhaps we can magically change by resonance in others.

Envision the person, thing, or situation that you are challenged by. Perhaps it is yourself, the person who gave you herpes, your diagnosis, or the challenges you face. Repeat these phrases five times as you imagine saying this to your subject:

I'm Sorry.
Please Forgive Me.
Thank You.
I Love You.

AFFIRMATIONS

- I love myself and my herpes because it shows me how to be compassionate to others.
- I love myself and my herpes because I know who is of value in my life.
- I love myself and my herpes because I am perfect as I was designed.
- I love myself and my herpes because I love and accept myself unconditionally.
- I love myself and my herpes because I forgive myself.
- I love myself and my herpes because I approve of myself.
- I love myself and my herpes because I am well-loved.
- I deserve all that is good. I release any need for misery and suffering.

This book is not all inclusive, and literature can change. It is important for patients to be seen by their medical provider and follow the medical advice of the provider.

Chapter Ten

CONCLUSION: MOVING FORWARD WITH VULNERABILITY AND COMPETENCE

"The reward for conformity is that everyone likes you but yourself."

— Rita Mae Brown

In this age, the life we live can be besieged by negative unhappy energy. To be able to get around that energy, we get to look at the positives. Life occurs as it happens and to play catch up can be difficult. It can be a challenge to have faith that this will work out in the end, but it has for me and it will for you. People in your life will take their cues from you. I have found that when I honored and loved myself, my family and friends could do nothing but reflect honor and love for me, too.

I am not necessarily proud of my actions in the years I did not fully disclose my history. I am, however, extremely proud of the person I have become since I decided to live authentically and in vulnerabilty. As a physician, I would like to educate you and influence others in a positive way through my own actions and lead by example. The truth is that herpes cannot be eradicated. It feels empowering to be integrated, honest, open and congruent. A positive outlook and sharing knowledge with others creates a positive culture.

Herpes can happen. It is grounding to know that you are created as perfect as you are, that you are whole by yourself for the rest of your life. You can overcome obstacles just by accepting yourself and being honorable and truthful. Struggle is common but for the life you want, it is worth it.

I encourage emotional balance in life. There is an emotional and physical component to herpes because stress, anxiety, depression can present as skin changes, high blood pressure, or constipation. This type of internal struggle that we feel can manifest in very obvious ways. It is not uncommon for me to have patients come into my office with certain ailments like pelvic pain, hormonal changes, and wonder how this occurred. It may just be simply from leading a life of incongruence. Be able to be good to yourself and be authentic. As human beings, we really like to know what is going on, but to control and manipulate others by hiding pertinent information for their health is unfair. It is a violation of ourselves as connected human beings.

As an obstetrician/gynecologist in the office and on labor and delivery, I witness daily woman's wonderful capacity to build loving, supportive families. Protecting loved ones and unending mental strength seems to be an innate trait. While it does seem easier to give into feelings of self doubt and back down from challenges, strong powerful women rise to the challenge, in my case, in their own time. Consider being a champion for herpes in your community and create a safe environment for women (and men) to share being herpes positive. This seed can grow and flourish into a community of people who begin to feel comfortable sharing their diagnosis and educating others. These once secret societies can normalize herpes into mainstream culture. Borders of these larger communities will coalesce and become influential to eliminate the stigma. I can be a cheerleader at the forefront, but your assistance will give more force to the movement. It is astounding to realize that we have herpes and we are not alone. Today is a new beginning, it can be that simple.

"There are no butterfly experts among caterpillars." One of my favorite Julien quotes exhibits the process of disintegration and reintegration. On a biological level, a caterpillar in its cocoon completely disintegrates and reforms into an entirely new living existence as a beautiful butterfly. On another level, a person can choose to be either the caterpillar or butterfly. The only way to understand being a butterfly is to become one. You have the power to become a better being. Embrace yourself, embrace what happens to you because in the end, life is juicy and fantastic. If I could hug my 20-year-old self and show her my influential path now, 15 years later, she would be so proud to say, "Yes, I Have Herpes, Too."

ABOUT THE AUTHOR

Raised in San Jose, California Dr. Sheila Loanzon completed an undergraduate degree in Biochemistry at Vassar College in Poughkeepsie, New York in 2002. Shortly after graduation, she traveled as a Delegate to the International Mission on Medicine to China based on academic achievement, leadership ability, and dedication to the medical profession. During this short four-week course, Traditional Chinese Medicine taught the governing philosophy that the body is whole, intimately connected, and has the potential to cure its own diseases. Dr. Loanzon discovered that nontraditional medicine and Western medicine should exist side by side, as both have their advantages, and thus her interest in osteopathic medicine began.

Dr. Loanzon graduated medical school in 2007 from Western University-College of Osteopathic Medicine of the Pacific in Pomona, California and completed an Obstetrics and Gynecology residency at Saint Francis Hospital in Evanston, Illinois, graduating as Chief Resident. In 2011, she joined a large multispecialty medical group performing complicated gynecologic surgeries as part of the select, minimally invasive surgical team, growing a full practice with beloved patients, and delivering care in the office and in Labor and Delivery.

Her interest in obstetrics and gynecology melds intellectual challenge, confined continuity of care, and comprehensive surgical and medical care for women from childbearing age through the postmenopausal years. Her goal is to provide tailored, effective medical attention to women in need.

CPSIA information can be obtained
at www.ICGtesting.com
Printed in the USA
LVOW11s1334080317

526545LV00004B/225/P